Contents

Colour plate section appears between pages 86 and 87

Clinicians' Guide to Epilepsy

Prefix
MTW

Clinicians' Guide to Epilepsy

P.E.M. Smith
S.J. Wallace
University Hospital of Wales
Cardiff
Wales
UK

A member of the Hodder Headline Group
LONDON
Co-published in the United States of America by
Oxford University Press Inc., New York

First published in Great Britain in 2001 by
Arnold, a member of the Hodder Headline Group,
338 Euston Road, London NW1 3BH

http://www.arnoldpublishers.com

Co-published in the United States of America by
Oxford University Press Inc.,
198 Madison Avenue, New York, NY10016
Oxford is a registered trademark of Oxford University Press

Whilst the advice and information in this book are believed to be true and
accurate at the date of going to press, neither the authors nor the publisher
can accept any legal responsibility or liability for any errors or omissions
that may be made. In particular (but without limiting the generality of the
preceding disclaimer) every effort has been made to check drug dosages;
however, it is still possible that errors have been missed. Furthermore,
dosage schedules are constantly being revised and new side-effects
recognized. For these reasons the reader is strongly urged to consult the
drug companies' printed instructions before administering any of the drugs
recommended in this book.

British Library Cataloguing in Publication Data
A catalogue record for this book is available from the British Library

Library of Congress Cataloging-in-Publication Data
A catalog record for this book is available from the Library of Congress

ISBN 0 340 76293 4 (pb)

1 2 3 4 5 6 7 8 9 10

Commissioning Editor: Aileen Parlane
Production Editor: Rada Radojicic
Production Controller: Martin Kerans

Typeset in 11 on 13 pt Garamond by Cambrian Typesetters, Frimley, Surrey
Printed and bound in Malta by Gutenberg Press

What do you think about this book? Or any other Arnold title?
Please send your comments to feedback.arnold@hodder.co.uk

Preface

General practitioners, general physicians and even neurologists who do not take a special interest in epilepsy often find the diversity of this subject confusing. For the paediatrician, the need to know about age-related syndromes and their specific managements and prognoses presents a challenge, which is often ignored.

This text aims to provide essential information in a readily accessible form. It is a book for the practising doctor who needs succinct and clear statements relating to the day-to-day management of the patient with epilepsy. The terms used in epileptology are defined. The incidence and prevalence of the epilepsies are considered both as a whole and for specific syndromes. Possible diagnostic pitfalls are examined from the newborn period to old age. In association with the classification of epileptic seizures and syndromes, the clinical features of the epilepsies are detailed. Appropriate investigations are discussed, with regard to both their choice and their timing.

Management is viewed in the widest sense: drug therapy, surgery, vagus nerve stimulation, diets, aromatherapy and relaxation treatment are considered, and the importance of the social aspects of epilepsy is emphasized. There are sections on seizures in the neonate and infant, and on epilepsy in the child and adolescent, in women and in the elderly. Learning and psychiatric disorders are reviewed, with some comments on non-epileptic attack disorder. The features relating to school, driving, employment, alcohol and mortality are given individual sections.

References within the text have been kept to a minimum; a list of useful sources for further reading is appended.

Acknowledgements

We thank the staff of the EEG department, University Hospital of Wales for printing the EEG figures. We are grateful to Pat Havard and Ceri Terrington for their secretarial help.

List of abbreviations

ACTH	Adrenocorticotrophic hormone
ADNFLE	Autosomal dominant nocturnal frontal lobe epilepsy
BECTS	Benign epilepsy of childhood with centrotemporal spikes
CT	Computed tomography
DNET	Dysembryoplastic neuroepithelial tumour
DRPLA	Dentato-rubro-pallido-luysian atrophy
DVLA	Driver and Vehicle Licensing Agency
ECG	Electrocardiogram
EEG	Electroencephalogram
EMA	Eyelid myoclonia with absences
GABA	Gamma-amino butyric acid
JME	Juvenile myoclonic epilepsy
MEG	Magnetoencephalography
MELAS	Mitochondrial myopathy, encephalopathy, lactic acidosis, and stroke-like episodes
MERRF	Myoclonus epilepsy with ragged-red fibres
MRI	Magnetic resonance imaging
NEAD	Non-epileptic attack disorder
PET	Positron emission tomography
REM	Rapid eye movement
SMEI	Severe myoclonic epilepsy in infants
SPECT	Single photon emission computed tomography
SUDEP	Sudden unexplained death in epilepsy
TIA	Transient ischaemic attack
VDU	Visual display unit

Introduction

Epilepsy

Epilepsy is a common and disabling disorder. For many people, it is a chronic and lifelong problem. The clinical features and underlying causes are very varied, and the classification of the epilepsies is still being modified.

For many years, epilepsy had been considered a straightforward but rather dull subject. A range of new treatments and the development of new diagnostic methods in the past 20 years have, however, revolutionized traditional thinking. A rapidly evolving understanding of the biochemical, structural and genetic abnormalities underlying the seizure tendency has spotlighted epileptology as one of the most exciting and interesting areas of medicine.

Epilepsy is not a single disease but is the manifestation of many possible underlying disorders. The rational management of any such chronic symptom depends upon a clear understanding of the underlying condition in a particular individual.

Epidemiology

Epilepsy is the most common of the serious neurological disorders. In a population of 10 000, a typical general practice, there will be 50–100 individuals with active epilepsy (a prevalence of 0.5–1 per cent), with four or five new cases arising each year (an annual incidence of 0.04–0.05 per cent) (Sander and Shorvon, 1996). The chance of any individual developing a seizure by his or her mid-70s (the cumulative lifetime incidence) is as high as 10 per cent (Hauser *et al.*, 1996); 4 per cent have isolated unprovoked seizures, and 3 per cent will have recurring unprovoked seizures (epilepsy). The discrepancy between these figures and the annual incidence emphasizes the temporary nature of epilepsy in the majority of cases.

The incidence of epilepsy follows a U-shaped curve in relation to age. The highest incidences are in childhood and in the elderly, reflecting the variety of disorders that may alter brain function in these age groups. The average annual incidence in childhood is 0.75 per cent, remaining stable during much of adulthood (0.3 per cent) and then showing a steep rise beyond 60 years, the annual incidence in the 80–84-year age group being 1.3 per cent (Hauser and Annegers, 1993).

A single seizure is, by definition, not epilepsy. Nevertheless, the chance of recurrence of a spontaneous single seizure has been shown, in a community-based prospective study, to be much higher than had previously been believed – around 70 per cent over the following year and 80 per cent over 3 years (Hart *et al.*, 1990). The recurrence rate following a single seizure is higher in those under 16 or over 60 years. There is a greater risk of recurrence following a partial than following a generalized seizure.

Social burden

Epilepsy itself can result in significant social handicap and exclusion, particularly as a result of educational underachievement, unemployment and inability to drive. The parents of children with epilepsy can have difficulty with delegating care to relatives or friends. These factors very often are as important to the patient and the family as are the seizures themselves.

Changing attitudes

Ignorance is the usual reason for the continued social stigma and for discrimination against people with epilepsy. Doctors' attitudes to seizure control are changing. Physicians have previously considered occasional seizures to represent satisfactory control but it is increasingly being recognized that the only truly acceptable outcome is complete freedom from seizures, since only then can there be freedom from the handicap associated with epilepsy. Only with good seizure control can there be normal psychosocial functioning, employment prospects and restored driving privileges. Occasional seizures may be tolerated in mainstream educational settings, but they are likely to cause secondary emotional and social problems and, if persistent, perpetuate the difficulties into adulthood.

Global perspective

Worldwide, epilepsy treatment is sometimes grossly inadequate. Despite the low cost of anti-epileptic medication such as phenobarbitone, nearly three-quarters of the 40 million people with epilepsy in the world are untreated. This extraordinary statistic is mainly the result of social rather than economic reasons. In many African countries, for example, there are prevalent misplaced beliefs that epilepsy is not physical but supernatural (evil spirits or witchcraft). As a result, most Africans do not seek medical help, believing that traditional healers are more appropriate for treating their disorder (Ahmad, 2000). Even in developed countries, a significant minority of people consider epilepsy to be a mental disorder (Kale, 1998). The first aim of any global campaign to improve epilepsy care must be to overcome the myths, misconceptions and superstitions surrounding epilepsy, and to increase awareness that epilepsy is a treatable brain disorder.

Epilepsy services

The diverse aspects of care dictate that epilepsy services must be multi-professional. It is important to give equal emphasis not just to the medical management of the epilepsy itself, but also to the social aspects. This includes considering the impact of epilepsy upon the individual, the family, school, work and place in the community. Such is the impact of these factors that a clear need remains for patient education, counselling and support, even when the seizures are controlled. Increasingly, the specialist nurse in epilepsy has helped to improve management.

Recent advances

Recent years have seen major advances in the understanding and management of epilepsy. Work at the cellular and molecular level has resulted in a greatly improved knowledge of the basic mechanisms of epilepsy. The immense challenge of unravelling the genetic basis for many of the forms of epilepsy is well under way. Better diagnostic methods have enhanced our ability to distinguish epilepsy from other forms of blackout, especially syncope and non-epileptic behaviour disorder. Advances in cerebral imaging methods can more precisely localize the sources of seizure discharges, with a view to potential surgical cure.

A widened choice of effective anti-epileptic medication has, for many patients, greatly enhanced seizure control and quality of life. The special issues relating to the management of epilepsy in childhood and in pregnancy have continued to develop. Epilepsy is widely recognized as a heterogeneous condition for which the most successful treatments are those tailored to a particular seizure type or epileptic syndrome: the evolving classification of seizures and epileptic syndromes reflects these advances and will enhance our ability to target treatment appropriately.

The classification of seizures and epilepsies

Introduction

The terms 'seizure' and 'epilepsy' are not synonymous. A seizure is a non-specific symptom with many possible causes, whereas epilepsy is an ongoing liability to develop that symptom.

What is a seizure?

A seizure is a stereotyped episode of sudden onset that may manifest as a disturbance of consciousness, behaviour, emotion or motor, sensory or autonomic function. It may be perceived by the patient, by an observer, or by both. On clinical grounds, it may be assumed to have resulted from an abnormal, self-limiting, paroxysmal or excessive discharge of a group of cerebral neurones. The definition is essentially clinical rather than based upon investigation results.

The correct classification of seizure types is very important as decisions on treatment and investigation depend upon their accurate identification.

What is epilepsy?

Epilepsy is a chronic condition characterized by a tendency to develop recurrent unprovoked seizures. Two or more spontaneous epileptic seizures occurring more than 24 hours apart are needed to fulfil this definition. Provoked seizures, febrile seizures and neonatal seizures are not considered to constitute a diagnosis of epilepsy. One episode of status epilepticus counts only as a single event, and so alone is not epilepsy.

The classification of epilepsy type and the recognition of epilepsy syndromes (*see* below) are essential in defining the probable aetiology, prognosis and appropriate treatment of an individual's epilepsy.

Classification of seizures

Seizures are classified predominantly upon clinical rather than electrophysiological information:

- **Partial or generalized.** Partial seizures are thought to have begun in a localized area of the brain, whereas generalized seizures are thought to arise in deeper central structures, involving all of the brain at once. In general, an aura precedes partial seizures, whereas generalized seizures occur without warning.
- **Simple or complex.** Consciousness is either retained (simple) or altered (complex) during a partial seizure.
- **Provoked or unprovoked.** Provoked (acute symptomatic) seizures occur at the time of acute systemic or central nervous system insults, for example associated with fever, metabolic disturbances, eclampsia or alcohol withdrawal, or in the first week after a head injury. For a diagnosis of epilepsy, however, there must be a propensity to unprovoked seizures.
- **Single or recurrent episodes.** A single (isolated) episode is defined as one or more epileptic seizures occurring in a single 24-hour period. An episode of status epilepticus counts as a single event. Two or more unprovoked seizures separated by 24 hours are required for a diagnosis of epilepsy.

GENERALIZED SEIZURES

In a (primary) generalized seizure, the symptoms and/or witness description give no indication of an anatomical localization for the seizure.

The five major types of generalized seizure are as follows:

- absence
- myoclonic
- generalized tonic-clonic
- tonic
- atonic.

Absence seizures

Typical absence seizures

Typical absence seizures in childhood present with a sudden loss of awareness without a total loss of posture. They may be associated with mild, clonic components, an increase in postural tone, a diminution in posture and automatisms (Penry *et al.*, 1975). About 40 per cent of absences have more than one component. The onset and offset are both abrupt, and the child is not aware that an absence has occurred. Typical absence seizures are associated with 3 Hz generalized spike-wave discharges on EEG (Fig. 2.1). This is

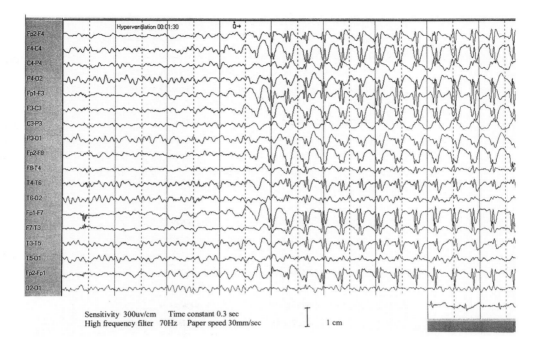

Sensitivity 300uv/cm   Time constant 0.3 sec
High frequency filter 70Hz   Paper speed 30mm/sec   1 cm

useful in distinguishing them from atypical absences (*see* below) or complex partial seizures (with localized seizure onset).

Atypical absence seizures

Atypical absence seizures are less well defined than the so-called 'typical' or 'classical' absences (Commission on Classification and Terminology of the International League Against Epilepsy, 1989). The clinical manifestations are comparable, although atypical absences tend to be less obviously abrupt in onset and offset, and consciousness may be clouded rather than totally lost. Atypical absences can be very prolonged. The essential distinction between typical and atypical absences lies with the EEG appearances. Atypical absences are not associated with 3 Hz spike-wave discharges but with other types of ictal changes. Slow spike-wave (less than 2.5 Hz) or fast activity usually accompanies atypical absences. Atypical absences are but one of several seizure types seen in the more severe childhood epilepsies. They occur particularly in the Lennox–Gastaut syndrome, in the syndrome of electrical status epilepticus during slow wave sleep, and in the more severe forms of myoclonic astatic epilepsy.

Myoclonic seizures

Myoclonic seizures have special implications for treatment. Most people are familiar with the normal (non-seizure) phenomenon of a generalized body

Figure 2.1
EEG: 3 Hz spike and wave activity, typical of childhood absence epilepsy.

jerk (myoclonus) occurring during light sleep. Myoclonic seizures are characterized by similar involuntary jerks, usually symmetrical and often occurring several at a time, each lasting a second or two. Consciousness is typically retained during myoclonic jerking. When jerking precedes a generalized tonic-clonic convulsion, it may be confused with a focal seizure onset.

Idiopathic myoclonic epilepsies

In idiopathic epilepsies such as juvenile myoclonic epilepsy, myoclonic seizures manifest as a sudden extensor jerking of both arms, characteristically occurring on or shortly after awakening, during which the patient typically may spill a drink at the breakfast table.

Symptomatic myoclonic epilepsies

More serious symptomatic generalized epilepsies also present with myoclonic seizures. In childhood, seizures presenting in association with metabolic disorders are commonly myoclonic.

Generalized tonic-clonic seizures

The tonic-clonic seizure forms the popular conception of a seizure. Typically, loss of consciousness precedes the 'tonic' phase (brief limb flexion followed by extension, often with a cry); this is in turn followed by the 'clonic' phase in which repetitive limb jerking gradually replaces the tonic contraction. The spasms often involve the whole body and are associated with tongue biting and other injury, frothing at the mouth, cyanosis and incontinence of urine or faeces. Patients typically are drowsy and confused with headache and muscle aching afterwards, sometimes for several hours.

The tonic-clonic seizure represents the end manifestation of a variety of initial seizure types, for example seizures generalized from the start or the generalization of a partial seizure.

Tonic seizures

Tonic seizures involve stiffening of the limbs and trunk followed by a fall, often with injury.

Atonic seizures

Atonic (astatic) seizures are associated with a sudden loss of muscle tone with a resultant fall, very often causing injury. In many cases, they are a limited form of myoclonic seizure.

PARTIAL SEIZURES

A seizure is partial if there is clinical evidence of a seizure onset that is localized to one part of the brain, regardless of whether it subsequently involves the remainder of the brain. The symptoms and signs depend upon the region of the brain in which the seizures arise; they include not just motor or sensory symptoms (e.g. from the frontal or parietal lobe), but also autonomic, psychic and cognitive features (e.g. from the temporal lobe) or visual symptoms (occipital lobe). The motor phenomena of a seizure may include automatic behaviours (automatisms), such as lip smacking, plucking at clothing, wandering, and so on.

The initial seizure symptom, the aura, is of important localizing value. Partial onset symptoms originating from various sites in the brain give rise to characteristic symptoms:

- **Temporal lobe seizures** are associated with epigastric discomfort ('butterflies'), déjà vu, a smell or a taste.
- **Frontal lobe seizures** are associated with adversive head turning, jerking of a limb or speech arrest. They are often nocturnal.
- **Parietal lobe seizures** are associated with lateralized sensory symptoms, such as tingling or pain.
- **Occipital lobe seizures** are associated with elementary visual hallucinations (colours and shapes) in the contralateral visual field (Plate 1).

Depth electrode EEG recording has, however, demonstrated that seizure symptoms can be very unreliable in localizing their site of origin. For example, falsely localized symptoms arise when some frontal lobe discharges are propagated through temporal lobe circuits during temporal lobe seizures.

Simple partial seizures

Consciousness is unimpaired during a simple partial seizure; that is, alertness and ability to interact with the environment are maintained.

Complex partial seizures

Consciousness is impaired during a complex partial seizure. Some patients appear alert and even speak normally during a seizure but afterwards have no recollection of the events. Altered consciousness should therefore include impaired memory for the event, as well as confusion or disorientation either during or after the seizure. The term 'complex partial seizures' is not synonymous with temporal lobe epilepsy since, although most originate in the temporal lobe, about 30 per cent arise from extratemporal sites, for example the frontal or occipital lobes.

Partial with secondary generalized seizures

A partial seizure may evolve to a secondary generalized seizure. This typically begins with an aura and progresses to a tonic-clonic seizure (*see* below). The aura is very important in classification. The progression to secondary generalization is sometimes so rapid that the seizure may appear clinically to have been generalized from the outset.

UNCLASSIFIABLE SEIZURES

In clinical practice, about one third of cases are unclassifiable, even after a detailed account from the patient and witness. If uncertainty exists, it is important not to be rushed into categorizing a patient's attacks since the management, including the information given about the prognosis and presumed aetiology of the seizures, will vary with the assigned seizure type.

PROVOKED (ACUTE SYMPTOMATIC) SEIZURES

Seizures occurring in close association with acute cerebral insults are designated 'provoked' seizures. Examples of provoking factors include metabolic disturbances, drug or alcohol withdrawal, and acute cerebral insults such as encephalitis, acute anoxia and head injury. Seizures occurring within 1 week of a head injury are considered to be provoked.

The management and prognosis of provoked seizures differ from those of unprovoked seizures. Management aims to remove the provoking factor; short-term treatment with anti-epileptic medication may be required, but long-term treatment is often not needed. The prognosis is that of the underlying condition.

NEONATAL SEIZURES

Seizures that occur in the first 4 weeks of life are likely to demonstrate subtle phenomena (*see* below); or be focal, or multifocal, clonic; or focal tonic or generalized myoclonic. Generalized tonic, focal or multifocal seizures may be rarely observed. Neonates do not have generalized tonic-clonic seizures.

Subtle phenomena recorded in association with EEG seizure discharges include ocular, oro-buccal and limb automatisms, autonomic changes and apnoeic spells (Volpe, 1995).

FEBRILE SEIZURES

These are epileptic seizures occurring in childhood after the age of 1 month that are associated with a febrile illness not caused by central nervous system infection, and occur without previous unprovoked or neonatal seizures. Such seizures may be generalized, or partial with or without secondary generalization.

STATUS EPILEPTICUS

This condition is characterized by repetitive or continuous seizures, lasting for at least 30 minutes. Any seizure type can keep recurring and thus constitute status epilepticus (*see* Chapter 6).

Spectrum of the epilepsies

The epilepsies encompass a vast spectrum of clinical presentations. At one extreme, the patient might be an otherwise normal adult with two previous minor sleep-related attacks requiring no specific treatment. At the other extreme, the patient might be a totally dependent, intellectually impaired child with frequent, intractable seizures of various types needing care and multiple interventions.

Classification of the epilepsies

A 'seizure diagnosis' (e.g. 'complex partial seizures') is made for most patients at presentation but merely describes their symptoms. It may help the choice of anti-epileptic medication but it does not imply aetiology or prognosis.

An 'epilepsy diagnosis' (e.g. mesial temporal lobe epilepsy) takes account not only of the main seizure type, but also of the probable aetiology, age of onset, neurological signs and investigation results (including EEG).

The classification of epilepsy is based primarily upon two factors:

- the **site** of seizure origin;
- the **presumed cause** of seizures.

In addition, syndromic classification is useful, particularly in children, since factors relating to neurological and cognitive status and probable prognosis are taken into account.

SITE OF SEIZURE ORIGIN

Epilepsies are classified into two major categories based upon the presumed site of origin of the seizures: localization related or generalized.

Localization-related epilepsies

Localization-related epilepsies manifest as a tendency to have recurrent partial seizures (with or without secondary generalization). Partial seizure onset might be suggested by an aura or by investigation findings, for example an EEG focus or a lesion on neuro-imaging. About 80 per cent of adult-onset and 60 per cent of childhood epilepsies are localization related.

Generalized epilepsies

Generalized epilepsies manifest as a tendency to have recurrent generalized seizures, i.e. seizures in which the first clinical changes suggest a simultaneous involvement of both hemispheres. Although essentially a clinical diagnosis, the ictal EEG patterns are initially bilateral.

PRESUMED CAUSES OF SEIZURES

Localization-related and generalized epilepsies may each be subdivided according to the presumed aetiology of the seizures (idiopathic or symptomatic/cryptogenic).

Idiopathic epilepsies

Idiopathic epilepsies are, in general, of genetic (or presumed to be genetic) aetiology. They are associated with normal intelligence, an age-specific onset of epilepsy, no obvious structural brain abnormalities and, despite seizure-related EEG discharges, a normal background EEG. The term 'idiopathic' (*idios* Greek = self) used to describe these epilepsies is traditional but slightly confusing. It does not mean just 'epilepsy of unknown cause'. In fact, the cause may be known precisely, given the knowledge of genetic abnormalities and gene products in an increasing number of 'idiopathic' epilepsies. It is, therefore, a special term reserved for epilepsies with particular clinical and EEG characteristics for which there is an implied or known genetic basis.

Symptomatic epilepsies

Symptomatic epilepsies have a known cause for the cerebral dysfunction, for example scarring, tumour or arteriovenous malformation. The term 'remote symptomatic' can be applied to epilepsies resulting from a long-standing static lesion, such as cerebral palsy (Fig. 2.2). A putative cause for all epilepsy can be found on clinical grounds in only about 25–30 per cent of cases. With very detailed investigation, however, this figure is much higher (Li *et al.*, 1995).

Cryptogenic epilepsies

Cryptogenic epilepsies are those localization-related or generalized epilepsies in which no underlying cause for the increased seizure risk has been identified but a microscopic structural cause is suspected.

EPILEPSY SYNDROMES

A syndrome is characterized by the co-existence of certain symptoms, signs and investigation results. For example, a patient with a certain epilepsy syndrome may have a characteristic age of seizure onset, have several seizure types, show characteristic EEG changes and may consistently show seizure remission at a certain age.

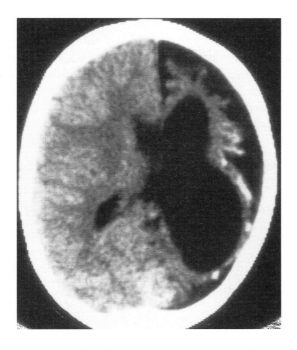

Figure 2.2
Computed tomography brain scan: long-standing left hemisphere damage with cerebral calcification in a man with hemiparetic cerebral palsy and hemiconvulsion epilepsy.

The major advantage of epilepsy classification stems from the recognition of epilepsy syndromes. This allows the clinician to:

- define the probable underlying aetiology of the epilepsy
- select the most appropriate treatment for that syndrome
- predict the prognosis for that patient's epilepsy.

Syndromes are not absolutely discrete entities, and two people with the same clinical syndrome do not necessarily have identical genetic or acquired disorders. However, as long as the causes of most epilepsies remain unknown, classification into syndromes is a useful way of characterizing symptoms and appropriately directing clinical management.

An epilepsy syndrome diagnosis might allow a meaningful prediction of treatment response, seizure-provoking factors and prognosis. Some diagnoses allow departures from epilepsy management conventions. For example in benign childhood epilepsy with centrotemporal spikes, one might not necessarily proceed to cerebral imaging following a simple partial seizure. Also, one would be confident in advising the parents that a remission of the epilepsy after puberty is almost guaranteed, as is the withdrawal of any anti-epileptic medication.

In juvenile myoclonic epilepsy (JME), one might begin medication after a single tonic-clonic seizure, continue treatment for life despite freedom from seizures, and even suggest maintaining valproate or lamotrigine, the treatments of choice for JME, during preconception and pregnancy (along with folic acid supplementation).

The ability to classify the epilepsies has advanced considerably in the past 10 years, and an increasingly rational classification will become possible as our knowledge of the molecular and genetic bases unfolds. At present, classification remains essentially clinical, based upon a recognition of patterns of symptoms and signs, and further refined by neurophysiology and neuro-imaging.

PROBLEMS WITH EPILEPSY CLASSIFICATION

Listing in age of onset order

Epilepsy syndromes are listed in the classification of the epilepsies (Commission on Classification and Terminology of the International League Against Epilspsy, 1989) in order of age of onset rather than frequency of occurrence. The classification of epilepsy syndromes therefore initially appears unbalanced, rare infantile conditions being listed first and the common adult epilepsies such as temporal lobe epilepsy listed last.

Unclassified epilepsies

A significant minority of newly diagnosed patients with epilepsy cannot be classified on clinical grounds alone (Manford *et al.*, 1992). The ability to classify epilepsy also depends upon the extent of the available history and investigations. The original classification was based upon clinical findings and EEGs; advances in cerebral imaging have meant that many epilepsies previously designated as cryptogenic can now be relabelled symptomatic. The finding of previously undetected but relevant abnormalities on high-resolution magnetic resolution brain scans in a high proportion of epilepsy patients (Li *et al.*, 1995) suggests that, with sufficiently detailed investigation, finding a defined cause of an epilepsy will become the rule.

The characteristics of recognized epilepsy syndromes are given in Chapter 3.

Other terminology

- **Active epilepsy.** A person with epilepsy who has had a seizure in the past 5 years has active epilepsy.
- **Inactive epilepsy (epilepsy in remission).** A person with epilepsy who has not had a seizure for over 5 years is in remission.
- **Catamenial epilepsy.** Catamenial refers to menstruation. 'Catamenial epilepsy' is the term applied to a cyclical change of seizure pattern with the menstrual cycle.

The clinical features of the epilepsies

Introduction

The epilepsies may be broadly divided into those which are idiopathic (presumed genetic) and those which are symptomatic or cryptogenic (with a known or suspected underlying cause). Some epilepsies are sufficiently well characterized to be assigned to a specific epilepsy syndrome, for example juvenile myoclonic epilepsy (JME). The clinical features of each of these groups are discussed below.

Idiopathic epilepsies

The idiopathic epilepsies are of presumed genetic origin, with normal cerebral imaging, often an age-specific onset and, overall, a good prognosis. Most patients with idiopathic epilepsies can be categorized as having an epilepsy syndrome. They can be broadly divided into those in whom seizures are generalized (idiopathic generalized epilepsies) and those in whom seizures are partial (idiopathic localization-related epilepsies).

IDIOPATHIC GENERALIZED EPILEPSIES

These syndromes are considered according to their age of onset.

Benign neonatal convulsions

Familial benign neonatal convulsions are dominantly inherited, most cases mapping to chromosome 20q and some to 8q (*see* Chapter 5). The onset is on day 2 or 3 of life. Short-duration attacks with tonic posturing and/or ocular symptoms are usual. Progression to clonic movements and gross motor automatisms, such as cycling, can occur. Remission occurs before 6 weeks in two-thirds of cases (Ronen *et al.*, 1993). Between seizures, the infants are well. About 10 per cent later develop epilepsy, characterized by generalized tonic or tonic-clonic seizures, which may be provoked, as in reflex epilepsies.

Non-familial benign neonatal convulsions show frequent clonic, often partial seizures, usually associated with apnoea. The onset is on day 4–6 ('5th day fits'). The seizures are sometimes repeated so frequently that status epilepticus supervenes. Remission nevertheless occurs over the following 6 weeks. The diagnosis is through exclusion, but once a diagnosis has been established, the syndrome has a good prognosis, only 0.5 per cent of infants having epilepsy later.

Absence epilepsies
(*See* Duncan and Panayiotopoulos, 1995.)

These syndromes are uncommon, comprising fewer than 10 per cent of childhood epilepsies. 'Typical' or 'classical' absence seizures predominate in five syndromes:

- childhood absence epilepsy
- juvenile absence epilepsy
- epilepsy with myoclonic absences
- eyelid myoclonia with absences
- peri-oral myoclonia with absences.

Childhood absence and juvenile absence epilepsies are the most common, and may well represent points on a single spectrum. However, childhood absence epilepsy is more common in girls than in boys (2:1), whereas the sexes are equally represented in juvenile absence epilepsy.

Childhood absence epilepsy
Childhood absence epilepsy has been defined as an epilepsy starting before puberty in previously normal children whose initial seizures are absences. The absences are very frequent, are not associated with myoclonus and are accompanied by synchronous 3 Hz spike-waves on the EEG (*see* Fig. 2.1) (Loiseau, 1992).

Incidence
The incidence of true absence epilepsy is difficult to determine from the literature because other types of minor seizure are often confused with absences. Cavazzutti (1980) reported that, among school-aged children with epilepsy, 8 per cent had absences.

Absence seizure types
Absences are usually brief, start and finish abruptly, are associated with a loss of awareness, with or without other changes, and occur many times, often more than 100 times, per day.

Penry *et al.* (1975) recorded 374 absence seizures by simultaneous video EEG in 48 patients. In 85 per cent of their patients, the absences were of less than 10 seconds' duration, and in all patients they lasted less than 45 seconds. These findings have been confirmed by later studies using combined video and EEG recordings.

There are six types of absence seizure. Individuals are likely to have the same type and duration of absences:

- **Simple absence.** There is an abrupt onset of complete stillness and loss of awareness, with the cessation of ongoing activities, but no loss of posture. The attack ends abruptly, and activity is resumed where it left off. Only 10 per cent of absences are simple.
- **Absence with clonic components.** The onset is abrupt. During the attack, clonic movements may occur in the eyelids (causing three per second blinking) or less frequently in other muscles, leading to rhythmic jerking, which is usually bilaterally symmetrical and does not impair posture. About 45 per cent of absences have clonic components.
- **Absence with increased postural tone.** Tonic muscular contraction may cause arching of the neck or back, which resolves before the end of the seizure. This is observed in only about 5 per cent of absences.
- **Absence with reduced postural tone.** A diminution in postural tone can lead to drooping of the head, rarely slumping of the trunk, dropping of the arms with relaxation of the grip, buckling of the knees and, rarely, a fall to the ground. Such changes occur during about 25 per cent of absences.
- **Absence with automatisms.** Automatisms during absences are of two main types. *Perseverative automatisms* are characterized by the persistence of an activity that was ongoing at the start of the seizure. *De novo automatisms* begin after the onset of the seizure and are characterized by licking, swallowing, scratching, 'fiddling' and other small-range, sometimes apparently semi-purposeful, movements. Automatisms during an absence relate to the duration of the seizure, being very rare in absences lasting under 3 seconds but present in 95 per cent of those of more than 18 seconds' duration. Automatisms are observed in about 65 per cent of absences.
- **Mixed absence.** In almost 40 per cent of absences, two (but rarely more) of the above additional components are seen.

Absences that are other than simple are referred to as **complex absences**. It can be seen from the above that the majority of absences are complex.

Absences can also be classified as **atypical** (*see* Chapter 2, p. 7).

Generalized tonic-clonic seizures occur in 30–40 per cent patients with absences, usually after the onset of the absences (Loiseau, 1992).

Clinical features

Childhood absence epilepsy is more common in girls than in boys (2:1). The seizures usually start in middle childhood between 5 and 10 years of age, but typical childhood absences may appear as early as 3 years or as late as 13 years.

Early authors considered that almost all children with typical absences were neurologically normal. Careful examination, however, often reveals minor difficulties with fine movement and coordination. Virtually all patients with absences are mentally normal. However, if absences are frequent, attention deficits are likely.

Using video-EEG with telemetry, absences have been shown to be less frequent in the afternoon than in the morning, and to occur less often in sleep (Nagao *et al.*, 1990). In rapid eye movement (REM) sleep and stage 1 of non-REM sleep, absences were as frequent as when awake, but in stage 2 non-REM sleep there were very few, and in stages 3 and 4 there were no absences. There is a significant inverse association between the duration of absences and their frequency (Nagao *et al.*, 1990).

Differential diagnosis

It is essential to distinguish childhood absence epilepsy from conditions that may resemble it clinically since the management and prognosis may be quite different. If possible, a seizure should be observed. Occasionally, video or ambulatory EEG monitoring is necessary to record a seizure.

Absences with automatisms may be difficult to distinguish from the complex partial seizures of temporal or frontal lobe epilepsy. The features helpful in distinguishing them are as follows:

- **Hyperventilation.** In the untreated patient, absences can almost invariably be precipitated by hyperventilation, whereas complex partial seizures rarely occur in these circumstances.
- **Post-attack confusion.** This is very unusual after an absence but almost invariable following a complex partial seizure.
- **EEG.** If the attacks cannot be distinguished clinically, the EEG, which is characteristic in absences, should clinch the diagnosis.

Children with **emotional difficulties** who become withdrawn or inattentive and those who are having problems with schoolwork are sometimes suspected of having absence epilepsy. Clinical and EEG observation during hyperventilation should resolve the situation.

Compared to typical absences, **atypical absences** are often more prolonged, less abrupt in onset and offset, and associated with clouding rather than loss of consciousness, and do not show 3 Hz spike-waves on the EEG. They occur in, for example, Lennox–Gastaut syndrome.

In **myoclonic absences**, myoclonic jerking of the proximal upper limbs is associated with loss of awareness (*see* below).

Aetiology

- **Frontal origin.** Absences are not usually associated with focal neurological deficits on clinical examination. Careful stereo-electroencephalographic work, however, suggests that the discharges originate in the mesio-orbital gyrus of the frontal cortex and are synchronized in the reticular system.
- **Genetic.** There is a family history of seizure disorders in between 15 per cent and 40 per cent of cases. Various modes of inheritance have been suggested, but the genetic contribution remains unclear, particularly in relation to the possible presence of a focal frontal lesion as the primary site of the epileptic discharge.
- **Febrile seizures.** In a population-based, case-control study, the only factor found to give a significant risk for absences was prior febrile seizures (Rocca *et al.*, 1987). Fourteen out of the 59 cases reported by Hashimoto *et al.* (1989) had had earlier febrile seizures.

Investigations

On **ictal EEG**, absences are associated with bilaterally synchronous and symmetrical rhythmic spike-waves. The discharges commence abruptly but cease over several seconds. Spike-wave complexes have a frequency of 3 Hz at the onset but may slow to 2.5–2 Hz towards the end of the attack. Irregular spike-wave discharges may also accompany childhood absence seizures (Loiseau, 1992). Generalized rhythmic delta activity may occasionally be associated with absences.

Between attacks, the background activity seen on the inter-ictal EEG is usually normal, but single or brief discharges may be found without any recognizable clinical accompaniment. Hyperventilation will usually precipitate an attack if the resting record is non-contributory.

Prognosis

In terms of seizures:

- **Absences** rarely persist beyond adolescence. Good prognostic factors are a rapid response to therapy, an IQ of at least 90, no history of generalized tonic-clonic seizures and no history of absence status.
- **Generalized tonic-clonic seizures.** About 40 per cent of children with absences later develop generalized tonic-clonic seizures, typically 5–10 years after the onset of the absences. They are usually infrequent and readily controlled by sodium valproate. The factors that increase the likelihood of developing generalized tonic-clonic seizures are the onset of absences after

8 years of age, male sex, a poor initial response of the absences to therapy and abnormalities of background activity and/or photosensitivity on the EEG (Loiseau, 1992). If the first seizures are generalized tonic-clonic, the outlook for remission is worse than if the epilepsy starts with absences.

- **Cognition.** Although intelligence is usually normal, absences that are inadequately controlled are associated with attention deficits and educational underachievement.
- One-third of patients have **behavioural problems** that are attributed to frequent attacks, to the effects of the parents' attitudes to the absences, or to therapy (Loiseau, 1992).

Juvenile absence epilepsy

The age of onset of this syndrome is around puberty, males and females being equally affected.

The seizures are clinically similar to those in childhood absence epilepsy but with important differences: they occur infrequently and often sporadically, retropulsive eye movements are less common during the absences, and they are associated with a less complete impairment of cognition (although some impairment of consciousness is invariable). Generalized tonic-clonic seizures nearly always occur, usually on awakening. Myoclonic seizures may also be present.

Spike-wave discharges on the EEG have a frequency greater than 3 Hz, usually 3.5–4 Hz.

Juvenile absence epilepsy does not remit, but absences may become less frequent after the age of 30 years.

Absence status epilepticus

The various types of absence status epilepticus (Shorvon, 1994) are considered in Chapter 6.

Epilepsy with myoclonic absences

This syndrome is characterized by frequent seizures in which clonic jerks are associated with 3 Hz spike-waves on the EEG (Manonmani and Wallace, 1994).

Incidence

Myoclonic absences are rare. Only 0.5–1 per cent of a selected population of children with epilepsy had this seizure type (Tassinari *et al.*, 1992).

Seizure types

The onset and offset of **myoclonic absences** are abrupt. Seizures occur frequently throughout the day and are of 10–60 seconds' duration.

Consciousness may not be completely lost, though it is impaired in most instances. The motor component consists of a rhythmic jerking of the shoulders, head and arms, and staggering. Falls are unusual. An arrest or alteration in the respiratory pattern may be observed. Some patients are incontinent during the attacks. A tonic contraction may follow the initial myoclonia.

Generalized tonic-clonic seizures are also seen in some patients. Hyperventilation will precipitate the attacks in about two-thirds of the cases, and about half the children are photosensitive. Wakening from sleep may also precipitate attacks.

Clinical features

Males are affected more commonly than females. The attacks may begin at almost any age during childhood. In about half the cases, mental retardation precedes the onset of seizures.

Differential diagnosis

- Myoclonic absences differ from other absences by the relative prominence of motor symptoms.
- Other syndromes with myoclonia tend to have 2 Hz spike-wave discharges on EEG rather than the 3 Hz frequency seen in this syndrome.

Aetiology

Epilepsy with myoclonic absences may be intermediary between idiopathic generalized and symptomatic generalized epilepsies. Genetic factors appear to be important. A family history of epilepsy is present in 25 per cent of cases; otherwise, nothing is known of the aetiology. Chromosomal abnormalities, for example trisomy 12p, may rarely be associated with this syndrome (Elia *et al.*, 1998).

Investigations

During seizures, the **ictal EEG** shows rhythmic 3 Hz spike-waves, which are bilateral, synchronous and symmetrical. The spike onset of the spike-wave discharge is strictly and constantly related to the myoclonic jerk.

Photosensitivity is demonstrated in about half of the children; attacks are provoked by hyperventilation in about two-thirds.

Treatment

A combination of sodium valproate and ethosuximide is most likely to control the seizures. Lamotrigine was effective in a small number of patients who failed to respond to ethosuximide, valproate or clonazepam (Manonmani and Wallace, 1994).

Prognosis

- **Seizures.** The seizures remit in some cases. In others, they become complicated by the appearance of tonic attacks and atypical absences such as occur in the Lennox–Gastaut syndrome. The EEG then shows slow spike-wave discharges rather than 3 Hz paroxysms.
- **Neurological handicaps.** Gross disturbances do not usually occur, but most affected children are mildly ataxic and some have moderate or severe dyspraxia.
- **Cognition.** Of the children who are intellectually normal at the onset of the myoclonic absences, about half later lose cognitive skills. About 75 per cent are finally intellectually impaired.
- **Behaviour.** No specific behaviour has been related to epilepsy with myoclonic absences.

Eyelid myoclonia with absences

Pooled experiences of a relatively small number of patients led to the description of this syndrome (Duncan and Panayiotopoulos, 1996). Eyelid myoclonia is associated with brief absences. The EEG shows generalized discharges of 3–6 Hz polyspikes and slow waves, usually of 3–4 seconds' duration, precipitated by eye closure, and photosensitivity.

Incidence

This syndrome is underdiagnosed, albeit admittedly rare. The incidence and prevalence are not known accurately, but possibly 5 per cent of children with absences have eyelid myoclonia with absences (EMA).

Seizure types

- **Eyelid myoclonia.** This consists of rapid and brief eyelid flickering with upward jerking of the eyes and head. Episodes occur many times a day and are associated with moderate impairment of consciousness.
- **Photosensitivity.** All patients are photosensitive; the sun or flickering lights can precipitate eyelid myoclonias.
- **Generalized tonic-clonic seizures.** Such seizures occur in virtually all patients, although they are very infrequent.
- **Limb myoclonia.** Infrequent myoclonic jerks of the upper limbs are unusual but reported.

Clinical features

EMA usually begins in middle childhood and persistence into adulthood is common. In some series, particularly those including adults, there is a predominance of females.

Differential diagnosis

The main differential diagnosis is **typical absence epilepsy**. The absences of EMA show an eyelid closure movement that is more distinctly myoclonic, rhythmic and random than is seen in typical absences. Consciousness may be impaired in EMA rather than completely lost as in typical absences. Ictal polyspike discharges are more characteristic of EMA than of typical absences.

EMA is sometimes misdiagnosed as **tics**.

Aetiology

Genetic factors are important, and there is a family history of epilepsy in most affected patients. No structural abnormalities are found on neuro-imaging.

Pathophysiology

No underlying pathological substrate has been identified.

Investigations

Electroencephalography is the principal test. Ictal clinical and EEG manifestations recorded by video-EEG show that seizures start with 4–6 Hz small-range myoclonic jerks of the eyelids with simultaneous vertical jerking and upward deviation of the eyes, accompanied by 3–6 Hz generalized discharges of mainly polyspikes and polyspike/slow waves.

Prognosis

- **Seizures.** Although EMA responds reasonably well to valproate, reports of the syndrome in adults suggest that control may not always be maintained.
- **Neurological handicap.** No specific problems have been identified.
- **Cognition and behaviour.** There are in general no major difficulties, although individual children may have educational and behavioural problems.

Peri-oral myoclonia with absences

This is a rare syndrome in which frequent typical absence seizures are associated with variable impairment of consciousness and localized rhythmic myoclonus of the peri-oral muscles (Panayiotopoulos *et al.*, 1994).

Seizure types

In addition to the absences with peri-oral myoclonia, all patients have generalized tonic-clonic seizures. These often precede the recognition of the absences. Absence status is more common in this than in other epilepsies with typical absence seizures.

Clinical features

The onset is usually in mid to late childhood or early adolescence, the absences tending to persist into adulthood. There are no cognitive or neurological problems and no behavioural difficulties.

Differential diagnosis

- **Absence epilepsy.** In absence epilepsy of childhood, consciousness is completely lost during the seizures.
- **Partial seizures.** These may also be confused with absences. Simultaneous video-EEG is helpful in these circumstances.

Aetiology

There is often a family history of epilepsy. No structural abnormalities are found on neuro-imaging.

Investigations

An EEG is mandatory in making the diagnosis. The **ictal EEG** shows high-amplitude discharges of spike, mainly polyspike, and slow waves at 3–4 Hz.

Video-EEG is particularly helpful. Peri-oral myoclonia consists of rhythmic contractions of the orbicularis oris, causing protrusion of the lips; contractions of the depressor anguli oris, causing twitching of the corners of the mouth; or, in more widespread involvement, myoclonia of the muscles of mastication leads to jaw jerking. Each myoclonic jerk is closely related to the polyspike component of EEG discharge.

The **inter-ictal EEG** may be normal or show focal spike or spike-wave discharges. Photosensitivity is not a feature of this syndrome.

Idiopathic epilepsies with prominent myoclonus

There are three main syndromes:

- benign myoclonic epilepsy in infants
- myoclonic–astatic epilepsy
- juvenile myoclonic epilepsy.

Benign myoclonic epilepsy in infants

Clinical features

Myoclonic seizures occur in infants who are otherwise neurologically and intellectually intact. The original descriptions of this syndrome suggested that it was a temporary epilepsy, unlikely to be of importance to older children. With better definition and recognition, it is, however, clear that some children continue to have seizures (usually generalized tonic-clonic) in later childhood. This is especially likely if valproate, which is particularly effective in this condition, is withdrawn (Dravet *et al.*, 1992). Thus, children with this syndrome need special consideration when the withdrawal of therapy is considered in later childhood or adolescence. If photosensitivity has been demonstrated, it is probably wise to continue with medication.

Prognosis

The categorization benign sometimes seems to be relative. School-age children who have had benign myoclonic epilepsy of infancy are likely to have an intelligence level within the average range, but many, if not most, have specific difficulties. They have often had specific speech and language difficulties, and many are dyspraxic. Their particular difficulties need assessment by skilled personnel.

Myoclonic–astatic epilepsy

Clinical features

Myoclonic–astatic epilepsy commences before the age of 5 years in 94 per cent of cases (Doose, 1992). Myoclonic and astatic seizures predominate, but generalized tonic-clonic seizures and atypical absences may also be seen. Since this syndrome can be somewhat resistant to drugs, continued myoclonic, myoclonic–astatic, absence and generalized tonic-clonic seizures may persist into later childhood.

Astatic seizures are undoubtedly the most disabling of the seizure types. A liability to sudden loss of posture is a liability to injury. Protective helmets may minimize head injuries in environments such as the playground. However, it is difficult to protect the child's face completely when, for example, eating hot soup, or to be on guard continually against a fall in potentially dangerous situations such as on a staircase. For these reasons, older children with myoclonic–astatic epilepsy often lead lives that are both physically and socially restricted. It is important to try to obtain freedom from astatic seizures, even if complete remission cannot be achieved.

Prognosis

A wide range of possibilities may follow the onset of myoclonic–astatic epilepsy. For some children, the condition will remit completely during middle to late childhood, with a good cognitive outcome. For others, seizures prove difficult to control, and there are significant cognitive, and therefore educational, implications. Most children with myoclonic–astatic epilepsy will need additional attention, either in relation to physical supervision, for cognitive problems, or for both, in the early school years. By adolescence, the long-term outlook should be clearer.

Factors suggesting a poor long-term prognosis include an early onset with generalized tonic-clonic seizures, the occurrence of periods of non-convulsive status epilepticus, and EEG changes of either the persistence of rhythmic slowing or the failure of development of a stable occipital alpha rhythm by the time of adolescence.

Juvenile myoclonic epilepsy

This is an important syndrome that comprises 5–10 per cent of adult epilepsies. It presents in the teenage years, but the epilepsy tendency persists for life. It is undoubtedly underdiagnosed, mainly because clinicians fail to ask specifically about myoclonic jerks in people presenting with seizures. The diagnosis has important implications for treatment since sodium valproate and lamotrigine are the recommended first choices; carbamazepine can potentially worsen the absences and myoclonic jerks.

Myoclonic seizures commence round about puberty, are particularly common just after wakening, and are often associated with photosensitivity. Infrequent generalized tonic-clonic seizures develop in most cases.

Juvenile myoclonic epilepsy is relatively common. Where video-EEG recordings are obtained from adolescents and adults, juvenile myoclonic epilepsy accounts for 12 per cent of all patients studied and 36 per cent of patients with various forms of generalized minor seizures (Wolf, 1992).

Seizure types and age of onset

There are three main seizure types:

Simple absences occur in about one-third of patients. They are often the first seizure type to appear, presenting between 5 and 16 years of age.

Myoclonic seizures occur next, between 1 and 9 years later, and are likely to be present before 15 or 16 years of age. They are bilateral, single or repeated, arrhythmic and irregular. They predominantly affect the arms; sudden falls with the jerks are unusual, and consciousness is usually retained. They are most likely to occur in the mornings on awakening and may be provoked by flashing lights.

Generalized tonic-clonic seizures also occur in most cases. The age of onset is usually after that of myoclonic jerks, but can be earlier. Again, they occur almost exclusively on awakening. Some patients are aware of precipitation of the seizures by flicker phenomena.

Clinical features

Males and females are affected equally. Myoclonic jerks begin in the early to mid teens. Neurological examination and intelligence are virtually always normal, but in one study of 10 cases there was mild dysfunction in two patients and severe dyspraxia in one (Clement and Wallace, 1990). Sleep deprivation, excessive alcohol intake, emotional stress and menstruation may precipitate the seizures.

Case report

A 16-year-old girl presented with her first generalized tonic–clonic seizure. She had been up at 5 am the day before and had revised for exams all day until 11 pm. As she rose from bed, she developed an involuntary 'jumping' of the arms followed by a loss of consciousness and a generalized convulsion. She bit the lateral aspect of her tongue, was incontinent of urine and was drowsy and disorientated afterwards.

On further enquiry, she reported that she had for 1 year experienced similar involuntary jumps of her arms, especially following sleep deprivation. They would occasionally cause her to spill drinks at breakfast time. Her mother had noticed occasional staring episodes, sometimes accompanying the jumps. Her inter-ictal EEG showed a normal background but with bursts of generalized poly-spike and wave activity.

She was diagnosed as having juvenile myoclonic epilepsy and prescribed lamotrigine, built up to a maintenance dose of 200 mg daily (together with folic acid 5 mg daily). She has remained seizure free on medication.

The myoclonic jerks are often not recognized as having an epileptic basis until a generalized tonic-clonic seizure occurs. The importance of asking about early morning jerks in an adolescent who has a generalized tonic-clonic seizure cannot be overemphasized since juvenile myoclonic epilepsy is in most cases a lifelong condition.

The inclusion and exclusion criteria for juvenile myoclonic epilepsy are listed in Table 3.1.

Enquire about early morning myoclonic jerks in any young adult presenting with a seizure.

Aetiology

There is a genetic predisposition to this syndrome. A positive family history of a seizure disorder is seen in approximately 25 per cent of cases; most affected family members have generalized seizure disorders. Some evidence links juvenile myoclonic epilepsy to genes located at chromosome 6p21.3 (Delgado-Escueta *et al.*, 1989), possibly associated with HLA DRW6 (Panayiotopoulos, 1996). Some families, however, show a linkage to chromosome 15q, and others show no linkage to either of these areas.

Pathophysiology

On clinical grounds, no particular underlying lesion or previous event appears consistently to predispose to juvenile myoclonic epilepsy.

Table 3.1
Inclusion and exclusion criteria for juvenile myoclonic epilepsy (Panayiotopoulos, 1996)

Inclusion criteria	Exclusion criteria
A predominance of myoclonic jerks and generalized tonic–clonic seizures; absences, if they occur, are mild	Clinical and/or EEG evidence that the myoclonia are secondary to brain hypoxia, metabolic disease or other structural brain abnormalities
A lack of neurological and/or intellectual deficit, while recognizing that juvenile myoclonic epilepsy may occur in patients with such problems, caused by other factors	Myoclonic jerks symptomatic of other epilepsy syndromes
The presence of generalized spike and/or multiple spike-slow wave discharges in untreated patients, while noting that treated patients may have normal EEGs	Generalized seizures, which might be tonic–clonic or absences, without definite evidence of myoclonia
Normal brain imaging where this has been performed	EEG abnormalities but no clinical evidence of seizures

Magnetic resonance brain images appear normal, but a more detailed analysis of magnetic resonance scans in juvenile myoclonic epilepsy has demonstrated a significantly increased volume of cortical grey matter compared with controls, suggesting a degree of cortical dysplasia (Woermann *et al.*, 1999). Microdysgenesis has been reported in the cerebrum of one patient (Meencke and Janz, 1984). Since intellectual deterioration does not occur, it seems likely that the seizures do not have serious pathological consequences.

Investigations

Ictal changes consist of paroxysmal polyspike and slow wave discharges. These are usually bilaterally synchronous and symmetrical, but there may be some inter-hemispheric asymmetry.

The background activity of the **interictal EEG** is almost always normal. Polyspike wave complexes also occur interictally, but these discharges have fewer spikes prior to the slow waves than when myoclonic jerks are observed.

Photosensitivity is more commonly demonstrable in this epileptic syndrome than in any other except EMA (Fig. 3.1). Patients also have polyspike wave discharge on eye closure.

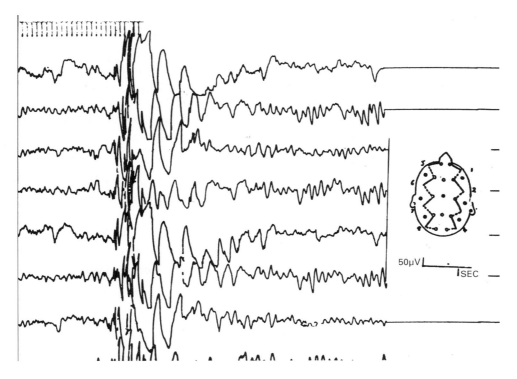

50µV

SEC

Prognosis

- **Seizures.** Although the seizures are usually readily responsive to valproate or lamotrigine, they tend to recur if treatment is discontinued. It is now recommended that anti-epileptic medication be maintained for life.
- **Neurological and intellectual status.** Neither new neurological disability nor intellectual handicap is likely to present in the long term.
- **Behaviour.** Immature personality traits have been highlighted, and poor social adjustment seems more common than expected (Clement and Wallace, 1990).

Figure 3.1
EEG: photoconvulsive response to 10 Hz photic stimulation (top left).

Idiopathic epilepsies with generalized tonic-clonic seizures as the main feature

Epilepsy with generalized tonic-clonic seizures on awakening

This relatively rare syndrome may be confused with juvenile myoclonic epilepsy if specific queries about myoclonic jerks are not made. Generalized tonic-clonic seizures are the sole manifestation and occur exclusively or predominantly shortly after awakening, regardless of the time of day. The age of onset can be between 7 and 35 years but peaks at about 17 years. Males are more commonly affected than females. Sleep deprivation is an important precipitant, particularly if associated with excessive alcohol intake.

The EEG may be normal, but increased slower frequencies, disorganized background activity with sharp transients and/or generalized spike-and-wave activity are more usual. Photosensitivity is very common. Neurological and cognitive functions are usually normal.

Valproate is most likely to control the seizures and probably needs to be continued indefinitely since withdrawal is associated with relapse in almost all cases.

Reflex epilepsies

Several factors may reflexly provoke epileptic seizures, but flickering light is by far the most commonly recognized stimulus. Seizures may, however, also be induced in susceptible people by pattern, by reading, or, very rarely, by games of chance, calculations and spatial decisions. If seizures always occur in very specific circumstances, consideration of a precipitating event is essential.

Photosensitive epilepsy

Photosensitive epilepsy is the most common form of reflex epilepsy and has become important because of the tendency for seizures to be provoked by television or computer games.

Incidence Photosensitive epilepsy occurs in 1 in 4000 of the general population, 5 per cent of all patients with epilepsy and more than 60 per cent of patients with visually induced seizures. The onset is usually in childhood between the ages of 4 and 19 years, but it is maximal around puberty. It generally improves with age in that at least 25 per cent of patients lose their photosensitivity during their 20s and 30s, although some remain photosensitive throughout life.

Diagnosis Most patients with photosensitive epilepsy can be diagnosed using intermittent photic stimulation on EEG. This involves using an electronic strobe light with different frequencies of flicker.

EEG In normal subjects, there may be a following (or driving) response – rhythmic activity over the occipital area limited to the duration of the stimulus. In patients with photosensitive epilepsy, there is a photoparoxysmal response (*see* Fig. 3.1 above) – bilateral generalized spike-and-wave discharges, usually outlasting the stimulus, which may be accompanied by myoclonic jerks or even a seizure (absence or tonic–clonic).

Mechanism Photosensitivity remains poorly understood but is presumably related to ineffective inhibitory mechanisms in the visual cortex and its connections.

Flashing lights   Seizures induced by flickering lights are usually generalized tonic-clonic, although they may be preceded by mild clonic jerking (Harding and Jeavons, 1994). Flash frequencies of between 15 and 20 Hz are most likely to be critical for the photosensitive subject. The age at the first seizure is usually in middle childhood, with photosensitivity apparently diminishing during the 20s, but not completely disappearing (Wolf and Gooses, 1986). In more than 90 per cent of patients, the stimulation of one eye is less epileptogenic than the stimulation of both eyes.

Discotheques   Most patients with epilepsy are not photosensitive. However, the incidence is highest in adolescents, the time of maximal exposure to recreational flashing lights. Photosensitivity is usually easily controlled on medication, and most photosensitive patients are prescribed medication. In general, therefore, discos do not need to be avoided. If a sensitive individual is inadvertently exposed to flashing lights, covering one eye often effectively prevents a provoked seizure. The greater danger for seizures at discotheques is from sleep deprivation, alcohol and recreational drugs.

Television   Thirty per cent of patients with a photoconvulsive response to intermittent photic stimulation are also sensitive to stationary patterns of striped lines (Wilkins and Lindsay, 1985). The most epileptogenic patterns are composed of stripes, subtend a large area of the visual fields, have a spatial frequency of between 1 and 8 cycles/degree, have a contrast in excess of about 30 per cent, have a high luminance, vibrate with a temporal frequency between 5 and 30 Hz in a direction orthogonal to that of the stripes and are viewed with both eyes. Television viewed at close quarters has just these characteristics. In Europe, the television monitor is the most common provocative stimulus for photosensitive seizures. This is because, in Europe, the basic frequency (refresh rate) is 50 Hz, whereas in most of the rest of the world it is 60 Hz. At 50 Hz, 50 per cent of patients with photosensitive epilepsy will show a photoparoxysmal response compared with only 15 per cent at 60 Hz. Popular, and particularly provocative, television programmes that include flash frequencies of between 10 and 20 Hz can precipitate seizures almost simultaneously in an alarming number of susceptible people (Fish *et al.*, 1994).

Video games   The advent of video games has highlighted a tendency to epileptic seizures in many individuals who otherwise had no evidence of a trait for epilepsy. Some people have photosensitive seizures only while playing video games, especially when playing for long periods. It is, however, the screen flicker rate (especially the 50 Hz refresh rate) rather than the content of the video game that is more important in inducing seizures.

Photosensitivity in epilepsy syndromes About 90 per cent of photo-sensitive patients experience generalized seizures (Wolf and Gooses, 1986). Childhood absence epilepsy, juvenile myoclonic epilepsy and the syndrome of epilepsy with generalized tonic-clonic seizures on awakening are significantly associated with photosensitivity. Photosensitivity is very unusual in the very young. Occasional patients with photosensitivity have only partial seizures, although in many of these the photosensitivity is found only on drug withdrawal.

Avoidance of seizures induced by intermittent photic stimulation
The following steps are recommended to avoid television-induced seizures:

- If possible watch television with a small screen.
- If watching a large screen, sit as far from it as possible (at least 2 m).
- View in a well-lit room with a light over the television.
- Use a remote control for switching on and off and changing channels.
- Use 'television glasses'. A sheet of polarizer to enhance the contrast of the picture is placed over the television screen. The patient wears polaroid spectacles in which one lens has an axis of polarization orthogonal to that of the other. The result is a functional monocular occlusion (Wilkins and Lindsay, 1985).

> Many patients with epilepsy wrongly believe themselves to be photo-sensitive and thus avoid flashing lights and VDU screens. It is therefore important to inform patients whether or not they are photosensitive.

Children and adults sensitive to patterns, sunlight on water and visual stimuli other than television should be taught to occlude the vision to one eye as soon as a potential epileptogenic circumstance presents itself. Many, however, find it difficult to comply with this suggestion. In some, there is a compulsion to view the television and other flickering phenomena at close and stimulating quarters, to the extent that they may deliberately light fires. Crossed polaroid spectacles may be helpful but are not always acceptable to the child. When physical methods fail, sodium valproate is the drug of first choice for the control of photosensitive epilepsy.

Primary reading epilepsy

This is a reflex focal epilepsy in which seizures are triggered by reading. They begin with myoclonic jerking of the jaw, mouth and throat, and, if reading continues, there follows a generalized tonic-clonic seizure. The EEG may show focal spike-and-wave activity over the left fronto-temporal region, or bilateral abnormalities.

IDIOPATHIC LOCALIZATION-RELATED EPILEPSIES

Most idiopathic epilepsies are generalized, but a few important syndromes are localization related. These are of presumed genetic origin and, despite a focal seizure origin, have no gross brain abnormality; they are associated with normal overall intelligence and a normal background EEG rhythm (Panayiotopoulos, 1999).

Benign partial epilepsies in infants and children

There are four main syndromes:

- benign partial epilepsy in infancy
- benign familial infantile convulsions
- benign childhood epilepsy with centrotemporal spikes (BECTS; benign rolandic epilepsy)
- benign occipital epilepsies (early and late onset).

Benign partial epilepsy in infancy

Infants have complex partial seizures and/or secondary generalized seizures but are otherwise neurologically normal. They show normal development, both before and after the period when seizures are occurring; there is no underlying neurological or other generalized disorder, normal interictal EEG and a good response to anti-epileptic treatment. A family history of comparable seizures is found in one-third of cases. The onset of the seizures is likely to be between 3 and 10 months of age. Remission occurs, on average, within 3 months but can be delayed for up to 12 months.

Benign familial infantile convulsions

It is not entirely clear whether this condition is completely separable from benign partial epilepsy in infancy. The onset is between 4 and 7 months of age. The seizures consist of an arrest of activity, a slow lateral deviation of the head and eyes, a loss of consciousness, diffuse hypertonia and unilateral clonic jerks that become secondarily generalized. Between seizures, the neurological, developmental and EEG status are normal. A seizure-free outcome, with normal neurological and cognitive development, is to be expected.

There is autosomal dominant inheritance, with some families linking to chromosome 19q or to chromosome 6. In the chromosome 6 families, some patients develop paroxysmal choreoathetosis, typically aged around 10 years.

Benign childhood epilepsy with centrotemporal spikes

Prevalence and age of onset

BECTS is the most common form of childhood epilepsy, with an age of onset of 7–10 years. It accounts for approximately 12–15 per cent of all epilepsies of childhood and is undoubtedly underdiagnosed. Seizures can start between 1 and 13 years, but the peak age of onset is 8–9 years.

Seizures

Two main types of episodes are recognized.

Simple partial seizures consisting of unilateral facial sensorimotor symptoms, oropharyngeal changes, speech arrest and hypersalivation occur soon after awakening. The affected child typically wakes the parents by arriving in their room first thing in the morning with facial asymmetry, an inability to speak and drooling. The attack is usually brief, but a unilateral clonic attack can supervene, with rare secondary generalization.

Generalized tonic-clonic seizures may present during sleep, either alternatively or additionally. These are likely to be of partial onset, but although the onset may not be witnessed, the child is often out of bed on the way to the parents' room at the time of generalization, suggesting some early knowledge of the attack.

Clinical features

Neurological examination is normal in the majority of cases, only minor asymmetries being demonstrable in the remainder. The overall intelligence is likely to be within the average range, but specific difficulties with literacy skills, attention and visuomotor tasks have been reported on detailed psychological testing. Transient cognitive impairment can be demonstrated during spike discharges. Occasional cases have serious linguistic impairment.

Aetiology

There are strong indications of a genetic tendency to BECTS, with evidence of linkage to chromosome 15q14 (Neubauer *et al.*, 1998). Prior personal and family histories of febrile seizures are common.

Investigations

The **EEG** shows characteristic changes. High-amplitude sharp and slow waves often occurring in runs are recorded from one, or very often both, central or mid-temporal regions (Fig. 3.2). A marked accentuation of the complexes occurs with sleep. If the awake EEG is normal in a patient suspected of having BECTS, sleep recordings should be obtained.

Neuro-imaging is normal in BECTS and is not indicated in cases considered

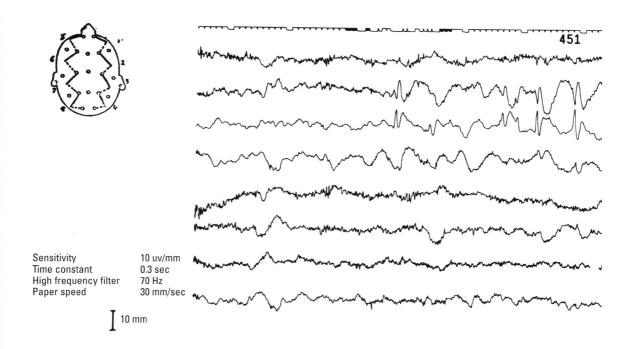

Sensitivity   10 uv/mm
Time constant   0.3 sec
High frequency filter 70 Hz
Paper speed   30 mm/sec

10 mm

to be typical. However, if there are any uncharacteristic features, magnetic resonance imaging (MRI) should be requested.

Treatment
The use of anti-epileptic drugs is not mandatory. If seizures are frequent, carbamazepine is the drug of choice.

Prognosis
The seizures almost always remit before or during puberty. Long-term learning, neurological and behavioural difficulties are not found.

Idiopathic (benign) occipital epilepsies
These syndromes are characterized by recurrent occipital seizures, EEG spikes or spike-waves abolished by eye opening, normal cerebral imaging and an age-specific onset. They are subdivided into those of early onset (mean age 3–6 years) and those of late onset (mean age 7–9 years).

Benign childhood epilepsy with occipital paroxysms (early onset)
(Panayiotopoulos syndrome)
This is the second most common age-related epilepsy after BECTS. The onset can be between 1 and 12 years, with a peak at 5 years.

The seizures are infrequent, usually nocturnal and associated with a deviation of the eyes and/or vomiting progressing to unilateral or generalized

Figure 3.2
EEG: right hemisphere centrotemporal spikes in a child with benign epilepsy of childhood with centrotemporal spikes.

convulsions. Irritability, pallor and wide opening of the eyes are common. Retching, coughing, speech arrest, cyanosis, oropharyngo-laryngeal movements and incontinence of urine are infrequent features. The duration may be brief, with resolution in a few minutes, or prolonged for hours. Spontaneous remission of the epilepsy is to be expected. The neurological and cognitive status is normal.

A prior history of febrile seizures is obtained in between one-sixth and one-third of cases. Family members have epilepsy in 7 per cent of cases, but forms of epilepsy other than Panayiotopoulos syndrome are likely.

The EEG shows paroxysms of occipital spikes occurring in runs on eye closure. If awake EEGs are normal, occipital spikes may sometimes be seen during sleep recordings. The spikes are seen maximally between the ages of 4 and 6 years. They may persist despite the remission of clinical seizures but usually disappear by puberty. No changes are seen on neuro-imaging.

Since the seizures tend to be infrequent and the epilepsy remits within childhood, the use of anti-epileptic drugs may not be necessary. If therapy is indicated, valproate and carbamazepine seem equally effective.

A seizure-free adulthood with normal cognitive and neurological skills is to be expected.

Benign childhood epilepsy with occipital paroxysms (late onset)

This is rare. The onset is between 3 and 16 years, with a peak at about 8 years.

Elementary visual hallucinations and/or blindness occur frequently when the child is awake and are characteristically very brief. The elementary visual hallucinations consist of small, multicoloured circular patterns, often appearing at the periphery of a visual field and becoming larger and multiplying as the seizure progresses; they often move horizontally to the other side (*see* Plate 1). Sensory illusions of ocular movements and ocular pain, tonic deviation of the eyes, eyelid fluttering or repetitive eye closure may occur. The seizures may progress to hemiconvulsions or generalized convulsions. During the purely visual phase of the seizures, consciousness is retained. Post-ictal headaches, which tend to be severe, unilateral, and indistinguishable from migraine, occur in one-third of patients. Rarely, orbital headache precedes the seizures. The neurological and cognitive abilities are normal.

This epilepsy is likely to be genetically determined since a family history of epilepsy, albeit usually of a different type, has been identified in about one-third of patients.

It may be difficult to exclude a structural cause on the grounds of the seizure type and the EEG findings. Imaging, preferably with high-resolution MRI, should be arranged. Where the EEGs show occipital paroxysms, these are precipitated in some cases by eye closure; in others, they are seen only during sleep. Random occipital spikes, or even a persistently normal EEG, can be found.

The seizures tend to be frequent and should be treated. Carbamazepine is the first choice and should substantially reduce the seizure frequency.

Approximately 60 per cent of patients will remit in late adolescence; the others continue to have infrequent seizures with visual symptoms and sometimes secondary generalization continuing into adulthood.

Autosomal dominant nocturnal frontal lobe epilepsy

This recently described syndrome (Scheffer *et al.*, 1995) may account for a significant proportion of patients with frontal lobe epilepsy. It is likely to be generally underdiagnosed as many milder cases presenting only with odd behaviour and restlessness in sleep may be erroneously labelled as familial parasomnias.

Patients with autosomal dominant nocturnal frontal lobe epilepsy (ADNFLE) present in childhood with predominantly sleep-related frontal seizures (*see* below). There is a marked variation in severity within families. Seizures include nocturnal tonic spasms, posturing and bizarre movements, often with retained consciousness, leading to a suspicion of hyperventilation or psychogenic attacks. Physical examination and brain scans are normal. The EEG may be normal, occasionally remaining so even during brief attacks. Carbamazepine is usually the most effective medication but many cases prove to be fairly resistant to medication.

Some families map to chromosome 20q13.2, the region coding for the neuronal nicotinic acetylcholine receptor α4 subunit (*see* Chapter 5).

Familial temporal lobe epilepsy

This autosomal dominant and relatively benign condition (Berkovic *et al.*, 1994; Wolf, 1992) has not yet been genetically characterized. Its main manifestation is as familial *déjà vu*, with little propensity for tonic-clonic convulsions. When secondary generalization occurs, it is usually nocturnal and following sleep deprivation or stress. The prognosis is usually good.

It is likely to be generally underdiagnosed since many cases with only minor attacks such as *déjà vu* perceive this to be normal for them (and perhaps normal for their family) and thus present only if they have a more major seizure.

Symptomatic and cryptogenic epilepsies

These are either generalized or localization related in type. Symptomatic epilepsies have a known structural cause (e.g. tumour or cortical dysplasia) whereas cryptogenic epilepsies have a suspected structural basis even though none has been identified on neuro-imaging.

SYMPTOMATIC AND CRYPTOGENIC GENERALIZED EPILEPSIES

These are the most disabling forms of epilepsy. Unlike other epilepsy syndromes, seizures are just one part of the illness, and not necessarily the major part. Associated problems might include the following:

- learning disability (mental handicap)
- challenging behaviour
- other neurological disability.

Symptomatic generalized epilepsy is often characterized by multiple seizure types and a resistance to medication.

There are many possible causes of symptomatic generalized epilepsy. Recent advances in cerebral imaging have demonstrated that disorders of cerebral development, for example lissencephaly or cortical dysplasia, underlie many severe childhood-onset epilepsies (*see* below).

Severe epilepsies with onset in infancy

There are four main syndromes:

- early myoclonic encephalopathy
- early infantile epileptic encephalopathy (Ohtahara syndrome)
- West syndrome
- severe myoclonic epilepsy in infants.

Early myoclonic encephalopathy

Myoclonic seizures start in the neonatal period. The EEG is characterized by suppression-burst activity. Inborn errors of metabolism are common: in particular, non-ketotic hyperglycinaemia has been associated with this epilepsy. The seizures respond poorly to anti-epileptic drugs. There is very little developmental progress, and death before the age of 5 years is usual.

Early infantile epileptic encephalopathy

Tonic seizures starting soon after birth are characteristic (Ohtahara *et al.*, 1987). The EEG shows suppression-burst activity, not readily distinguishable from that of early myoclonic encephalopathy but distinct from hypsarrhythmia (*see* below). There are many possible aetiological factors, most of which relate to structural brain abnormalities, usually of a prenatal, developmental origin. Seizure control is difficult, but lamotrigine can be helpful in small doses. There may be evolution to West, and later to Lennox–Gastaut, syndrome with continuing tonic as well as other seizure types.

Most affected infants survive to later childhood and early adolescence, but in severely handicapped states. Complete dependence is usual: immobility secondary to the severe cerebral state is complicated by joint contractures and scoliosis. Death from overwhelming respiratory infection is likely in mid or late adolescence.

West syndrome

West syndrome has three main characteristics:

- infantile spasms
- hypsarrhythmia on EEG (Fig. 3.3)
- developmental arrest or regression.

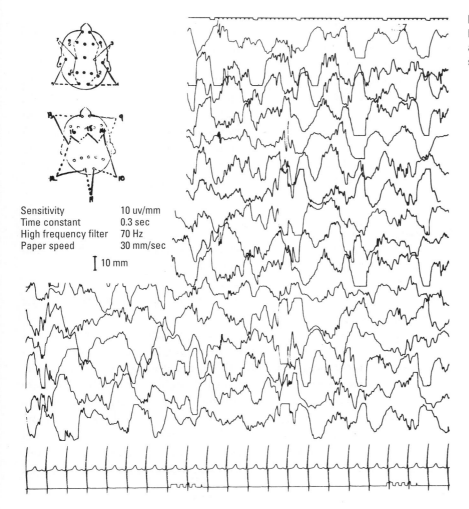

Sensitivity   10 uv/mm
Time constant   0.3 sec
High frequency filter 70 Hz
Paper speed   30 mm/sec

Figure 3.3
EEG: hypsarrhythmia in a child with West syndrome.

The original description was published in the Lancet in 1841 by a general practitioner who observed this epilepsy in his own son.

Incidence

Between 1 in 1900 and 1 in 3900 children develop West syndrome. The onset is virtually always in the first year of life.

Seizures

Spasms are the predominant seizure type. Each consists of a brief flexion, extension or mixed flexion/extension of the axial and/or limb muscles. Most commonly, there is flexion of the trunk and neck and extension of the arms. A brief cry may accompany the spasm. Spasms tend to occur in clusters, lasting about 10 minutes but often longer. Most spasms are symmetrical, but asymmetry may be observed.

Other seizures can be associated with the spasms of West syndrome: partial, myoclonic, tonic, tonic-clonic, akinetic, hemiconvulsive and atypical absence seizures have all been recorded (Plouin and Dulac, 1994).

Clinical features

To a large extent, the neurological features reflect the underlying pathology. Almost any type of physical handicap may be found. It is very important to consider whether the spasms are symptomatic of a genetic disorder. A full examination of all systems is essential. In particular, other stigmata of tuberous sclerosis should be sought. Cognitive difficulties are universal at the onset of West syndrome and persist in approximately 90 per cent of cases.

Aetiology

Almost any pathology that can lead to severe generalized brain dysfunction in infancy may be associated with West syndrome:

- **Cryptogenic.** A very small percentage of cases appear cryptogenic, the prognosis being much better for these.
- **Symptomatic.** When infantile spasms are associated with genetic conditions, these are usually dysplasias, for example lissencephaly, neuro-cutaneous syndromes (particularly tuberous sclerosis) or, rarely, metabolic encephalopathies. Dysplastic lesions, which are not obviously genetically determined, are common. West syndrome may follow hypoxic–ischaemic encephalopathy. Prenatal cytomegalovirus disease seems the most important of the possible infectious causes. Epidemiological studies have shown no association between West syndrome and pertussis vaccination. Chromosomal aberrations, such as Down's syndrome, may be complicated by West syndrome.

Investigations

- **EEG.** Hypsarrhythmia is one of the characteristics, manifesting as almost continuous high-voltage, slow activity with frequent, irregularly associated spike discharges (*see* Fig. 3.3 above). Modified or unilateral hypsarrhythmia can occur.
- **Computed tomography (CT) or MR imaging** must be requested since an understanding of the aetiology is likely to be helpful in both genetic counselling and prognosis.
- **Other tests.** In most cases, a full metabolic work-up and a search for evidence of prenatal infection are indicated.

Treatment

The main choice lies between vigabatrin and adrenocorticotrophic hormone (ACTH) (or steroids).

Vigabatrin controls the spasms in just over half of the cases and, in the short term, is less likely than ACTH/steroids to cause important adverse events. The peripheral visual field constriction frequently complicating the use of vigabatrin has, however, made clinicians wary of its use since treatment may need to continue for several years.

ACTH/steroids may also control the spasms, but ACTH in particular can render the infants hypertensive and liable to infection. For infants with an underlying structural brain disorder, the use of ACTH/steroids, in a course lasting up to 3 months, can produce only temporary relief.

Vigabatrin currently remains the treatment of first choice. For resistant spasms, high-dosage valproate, lamotrigine, benzodiazepines and pyridoxine are alternative or additional therapies.

Prognosis

- **Seizure prognosis.** Approximately 60 per cent of children continue to have epilepsies, usually with predominantly partial seizures. Some go on from West syndrome to Lennox–Gastaut syndrome, with prominent tonic seizures.
- **Physical handicap** relates to the underlying neurological problem and is common when infection or hypoxic–ischaemic encephalopathy is a precursor.
- **Mental handicap** is an almost universal sequel. About 90 per cent of the children will have global learning difficulties, and another 5 per cent have specific problems. Thus, only about 5 per cent are of normal intelligence.

The families of infants who develop West syndrome clearly require considerable support.

Severe myoclonic epilepsy in infants

Incidence

Severe myoclonic epilepsy in infants (SMEI) is one of the rarest forms of epilepsy. The seizures characteristically start with febrile illnesses, but only about 1 in 2000 children who have febrile seizures will later have SMEI.

Seizures

The seizure type evolves with age:

- In the **first year** of life, hemiclonic or bilateral clonic seizures occur in association with febrile illnesses. The clonic attacks may be repeated on several occasions.
- In the **second year**, myoclonia become evident, and tonic-clonic seizures (either of varying lateralization or generalized) and photosensitivity become prominent.
- In the **third year** and beyond, the epilepsy is characterized by the persistence of multiple seizure types and marked photosensitivity.

Clinical features

In the first year, the infants develop normally. The disorder usually becomes established in the second year. There is developmental arrest, with little, if any, further progress in cognitive skills throughout childhood. Physical abilities are less affected, although some degree of ataxia and the persistence of immature movement patterns are common.

The extreme photosensitivity may cause difficulty with management since children with SMEI tend to be transfixed by television and video screens, leading to further seizures.

Aetiology

No definite aetiological factors have been identified. Careful neuropathological studies have often demonstrated malformations of cortical development, particularly neuronal heterotopia.

Investigations

The EEG is initially normal during the time when clonic seizures with fever predominate. In the second year, as other seizure types develop, the EEG shows epileptic discharges, which are often to some extent lateralized. The early development of spikes and spikes-and-waves in response to photic stimulation should suggest SMEI.

CT and MR scans are usually normal. Underlying biochemical and genetic factors have not been identified.

Treatment

SMEI responds poorly to all current anti-epileptic drugs. Valproate is probably the most effective, but a complete control of seizures is very unlikely. Most children with SMEI will become worse if given lamotrigine, although this may rarely be helpful. Stiripentol, a P450 cytochrome inhibitor, is a promising new treatment.

Prognosis

Seizures continue throughout childhood despite treatment. Learning difficulties are severe. Affected patients remain dependent.

Lennox–Gastaut syndrome

This term is often loosely applied to any severe and refractory epilepsy of early childhood. There are, however, distinctive seizure and EEG criteria.

Incidence

Between 3 and 10 per cent of children with epilepsy have Lennox–Gastaut syndrome. The onset is usually between 3 and 5 years of age, and is very unusual after 10 years. There may be no previous neurodevelopmental problems, or prior learning and/or movement difficulties may be present; alternatively, the condition may evolve from West syndrome.

Seizures

- **Axial tonic seizures** occur in all cases.
- **Atypical absences** are common.
- **Atonic seizures** may be present.
- **Myoclonic seizures** are not observed in the purest forms of Lennox–Gastaut syndrome, but, in many children, it can be difficult to decide whether the epilepsy is Lennox–Gastaut syndrome with some myoclonia or a severe form of myoclonic–astatic epilepsy with learning difficulties. For this reason, some epileptologists feel that Lennox–Gastaut syndrome and myoclonic–astatic epilepsy are but extremes of a spectrum of severe polymorphic epilepsies of childhood (Aicardi, 1996).
- **Other seizures**, which are not typical of Lennox–Gastaut syndrome, for example tonic-clonic, clonic or partial attacks, are seen occasionally.

Aetiology

Lennox–Gastaut syndrome may sometimes follow West syndrome, or occasionally early infantile epileptic encephalopathy. Thus, Lennox–Gastaut syndrome may be secondary to any disorder leading to gross generalized cerebral disturbance in infancy or early childhood. Often, no aetiology can be identified. Pathological examination suggests that cortical dysplasias, especially neuronal heterotopia, are important factors. Genetic factors are not found.

Clinical features

The overall clinical picture is dominated by frequent seizures, which are usually difficult to control. Most children have neurological deficits. These vary in severity from mild pyramidal tract and cerebellar signs to moderately severe ataxia with plegias. Most are ambulant. A frank deterioration in locomotor ability is unusual, but the maturation of sophisticated motor skills does not occur. At the onset of the condition, there is developmental arrest; continuing learning difficulties are the rule. Most children have very limited expressive speech, but a few, who are less affected, read and write a little. Total dependence in adulthood is expected.

Investigation

- EEG. When awake, the EEG is characterized by 2–2.5 Hz spikes-and-waves. Thus, the spike-and-wave is of slower frequency than in typical absence epilepsies. Photosensitivity is not found. During slow wave sleep, widespread rhythmic spike discharges with a frequency of about 10 Hz predominate in the anterior areas. These are considered an important diagnostic feature of Lennox–Gastaut syndrome.
- **Neuro-imaging.** Imaging by CT, or preferably MRI, can define aetiological factors but is often disappointingly normal.
- **Other tests.** Metabolic and chronic infection screens are usually arranged but rarely give positive results.

Treatment

Complete control of seizures can be very difficult. A combination of valproate and lamotrigine is most likely to be effective. Somewhat variable results have been reported with vigabatrin. A course of steroids may terminate a bad patch of seizures. Benzodiazepines are effective, but tolerance readily develops. Much family support is needed.

Prognosis

Seizures are likely to continue despite medication. Learning, and to a lesser extent physical, difficulties restrict life activities very considerably.

Epilepsies with predominantly cognitive symptomatology

There is a group of epilepsies in which clinical seizures are relatively unspectacular but in which cognitive effects are predominant. Cognitive disturbance is the essence of the seizures, but brief twitches, changes in posture or colour, pupillary dilatation and other minor motor or behavioural changes are also likely to be present.

Landau–Kleffner syndrome

The features described in Landau–Kleffner syndrome, or epileptic aphasia, are now considered to be too limiting to take account accurately of the interferences with thought processes that occur. Nevertheless, the loss of first expressive, and later receptive, language abilities is an important component. The EEG shows diffuse changes with spikes and spikes-and-waves occurring randomly in time and space; temporal or parieto-occipital are more usual than frontal locations. In untreated or refractory cases, a loss of cognitive abilities tends to progress. Neuro-imaging is normal.

Epilepsy with continuous spike-wave discharges during slow wave sleep

This often co-exists with Landau–Kleffner syndrome. Again, clinical seizures are not prominent, despite a loss of cognitive skills and considerable EEG abnormality, especially during slow wave sleep. Neuro-imaging is again normal.

The treatment of these epilepsies can be difficult. Serial EEGs are often more helpful than clinical events in monitoring therapeutic effectiveness. Valproate, or valproate and lamotrigine, is most likely to be helpful. Vigabatrin has been reported to be effective in single cases. Steroids have also been used successfully. Multiple sub-pial transections (*see* Chapter 6) may be effective if a definite spike focus can be identified. In the long term, even if seizures remit and the EEG returns to normal, most children will have residual language difficulties, although these are of very varying severity.

Progressive myoclonus epilepsies

Dravet *et al.* (1996) have outlined the characteristics of the full-blown progressive myoclonus epilepsy syndrome:

- a **myoclonic syndrome** with a combination of fragmentary or segmental, arrhythmic, asynchronous, symmetric myoclonus and massive myoclonia
- an **epilepsy**, usually with generalized tonic-clonic or clonic seizures, but other types of seizures are also liable to occur
- a **neurological syndrome**, which nearly always includes cerebellar manifestations
- a **mental deterioration**, culminating in dementia.

Aetiology

There are a number of conditions for which progressive myoclonus epilepsies are at least a component. These may be classified (Dravet *et al.*, 1996) into conditions characterized by the following:

- a **biological marker**, such as in sialidosis type I, juvenile Gaucher's disease (type III), and myoclonus epilepsy with ragged-red fibres (MERRF)
- a **pathological marker**, such as in late infantile neuronal ceroid lipofuscinosis (classical and variant types), juvenile neuronal ceroid lipofuscinosis and Lafora body disease
- a **genetic marker**, as in the myoclonus epilepsy of Huntington's disease, Unverricht–Lundbörg disease and dentato-rubro-pallido-luysian atrophy (DRPLA).
- **no identified marker**, as in Alpers' disease.

They may be further classified by their age of onset.

Clinical features

Sialidosis type I This condition is otherwise known as the cherry-red spot myoclonus syndrome. It is an autosomal recessive disorder with a deficiency of neuraminidase (α-2-6 sialidase). The age at onset is usually about 15 years. Mild visual impairment, epilepsy and various neurological signs including cherry-red spots at the maculae can be present before myoclonus becomes an increasingly characteristic feature. Spontaneous, intermittent, irregular myoclonia of the face occurs which is not stimulus sensitive and persists during sleep. In the EEG, the background activity is normal or fast and of low voltage; massive myoclonia are associated with generalized polyspike-waves, but the facial myoclonia are not associated with EEG changes.

Juvenile Gaucher's disease (type III) Juvenile Gaucher's disease (type III) presents with myoclonus and saccadic horizontal eye movements, generalized or partial epileptic seizures, cerebellar impairment, dementia and sometimes splenomegaly. In the EEG, the background activity is normal or slow, and there are bursts of mainly posterior, sometimes multifocal, 6–10 Hz poly-spike-waves, which are enhanced by sleep. A myoclonic response is induced by photic stimulation.

Myoclonus epilepsy with ragged-red fibres MERRF is caused by a mutation in mitochondrial DNA and is therefore potentially maternally inherited. The main clinical characteristics are myoclonia, epilepsy and dementia, but many patients have other signs of mitochondrial disease such as deafness, optic atrophy, peripheral neuropathy and various endocrine dysfunctions. The seizures are tonic-clonic in type. The diagnosis can be aided by the finding of ragged-red fibres in the muscle biopsy (Plate 2), but confirmation has been made easier by the finding of the specific heteroplasmic A to G mutation in mitochondrial DNA.

Late infantile neuronal ceroid lipofuscinosis   The gene for this autosomal recessive disorder has been mapped to chromosome 11p15. Epilepsy, characterized by myoclonic seizures, is prominent. Dementia and ataxia occur soon after the onset, which is between 18 months and 4 years of age. Visual failure is associated with macular and retinal degeneration and optic atrophy. The EEG shows multifocal spikes on a slow-frequency background, with a very specific response to slow flash frequencies, when each flash produces a spike posteriorly. The electroretinogram is extinguished. Visual evoked potentials are of very high amplitude. Cytosomes containing curvilinear profiles can be found in skin or conjunctival biopsies. Death occurs in mid to late childhood.

Variant late infantile neuronal ceroid lipofuscinosis   This is an autosomal recessive condition for which the gene has been localized to l5q 21–23. In common with the more characteristic form of late infantile neuronal ceroid lipofuscinosis, the variant type presents with ataxia, a loss of acquired cognitive skills and early visual loss. The age of onset is, however, a little later; tonic-clonic and myoclonic seizures may not appear for a year or so, and the course tends to be more protracted.

Juvenile neuronal ceroid lipofuscinosis   Juvenile neuronal ceroid lipofuscinosis is characterized by an onset in late childhood or early adolescence of visual deterioration. Intellectual and other neurological signs appear within the next 2 or 3 years and epilepsy at a somewhat later date. The seizures can be absences or tonic-clonic initially, but clonic status can occur terminally. Segmental and late massive myoclonus appears coincidental with the seizures. The gene has been localized to chromosome 16p12. The diagnosis may be made on the finding of specific inclusion bodies, usually fingerprint membranous profiles and/or rectilinear profiles in biopsy maternal (skin, conjunctiva, etc.).

Lafora body disease   This condition is a rare autosomal recessive disorder, which starts late in the first or in the second decade. Survival is unlikely after the age of 30 years. Lafora bodies, deposits of polyglucans, are found in brain but may also be shown in skin, mucosa, liver or muscle biopsy material. Biopsy of the axillary skin is a satisfactory diagnostic procedure.

Generalized or partial epileptic seizures are usually the first symptom, followed by severe and progressive, erratic, resting and action myoclonus, and later by rapidly worsening dementia. There is a tendency for the symptoms to have periods of rapid worsening, with intervening plateaux. In the earliest EEGs, the background activity is normal, with isolated bursts of spike-waves and polyspike-waves, as well as marked photosensitivity. The epileptic paroxysms are not enhanced by sleep, nor are the erratic myoclonia associated with EEG changes. Months or years may elapse before the typical EEG pattern appears with slowing of the background activity, fast generalized polyspikes and polyspike-waves, focal occipital or multifocal spikes, the disappearance of physiological sleep patterns and persisting erratic myoclonus, with or without persisting photosensitivity.

Huntington's disease   Huntington's disease is characteristically a disorder of young to middle adulthood, chorea being the main clinical feature. Rarely, the onset is in childhood, when inheritance, always autosomal dominant, is from the father. The neurological symptomatology is very diverse in childhood, but rigidity, rather than chorea, predominates. Epilepsy occurs about 2 years after the onset, with tonic-clonic seizures, atypical absences and massive myoclonia. Photosensitivity may be demonstrable on the EEG even before seizures commence. Later, there are spontaneous bursts of spike-waves and polyspike-waves. The diagnosis is made by identifying an expanded trinucleotide (CAG) repeat at chromosome 4p16.3.

Unverricht–Lundbörg disease   This condition has been reported particularly from the Baltic and Mediterranean regions. There is an autosomal recessive inheritance, with linkage to a gene on the distal part of chromosome 21q22.3. The onset is between 6 and 18 years with either insidious action myoclonus on awakening or nocturnal clonic-tonic-clonic seizures. The myoclonia become incapacitating and can culminate in clonic or clonic-tonic-clonic seizures. Absences are less frequent. The ataxia is progressive. The intellect is always preserved, but the seizures, myoclonia and ataxia become very incapacitating. The background activity on the EEG is initially normal, with a few slow discharges. Short, subclinical spike-wave discharges become more frequent in the initial stages of the disease but tend to disappear later. Photosensitivity is almost invariably present.

Dentato-rubro-pallido-luysian atrophy   DRPLA is an autosomal dominant condition, associated with an unstable expansion of the CAG repeat in chromosome 12 and mainly reported from Japan. There is a very wide age range at onset, with some patients first affected at 6 years old. Progressive myoclonus epilepsy can be associated with choreoathetosis, dementia and ataxia. Bursts of slow activity and generalized spike-waves are seen on the EEG.

SYMPTOMATIC AND CRYPTOGENIC LOCALIZATION-RELATED EPILEPSIES

Symptomatic localization-related epilepsies follow localized central nervous system insults. If the disorder is localized to one area of the brain, the seizure type will be predictable from the lobe damaged and classified according to that lobe, for example as frontal lobe epilepsy.

If a localized central nervous system insult is suspected but not identified, the epilepsy is designated 'cryptogenic'. This is the most common epilepsy type in both adults and children. Temporal lobe epilepsy is the most frequently diagnosed. Most symptomatic epilepsies are not classifiable into syndromes. Nevertheless, syndromic features aid treatment decisions and the assessment of prognosis.

Temporal lobe epilepsy

This is the most common adult-onset epilepsy.

Causes

Temporal lobe seizures in adults are usually caused by pathology in the mesial temporal area.

Mesial temporal sclerosis is the most common cause. Here, there is gliosis or scarring of one or both hippocampi, which is thought to develop very early in life, perhaps in association with febrile convulsions (*see* below) (Fig. 3.4).

Rarer causes are tumours (including ganglioglioma and dysembryoplastic neuroepithelial tumour (Fig. 3.5), cavernoma and abnormal neuronal migration (*see* below).

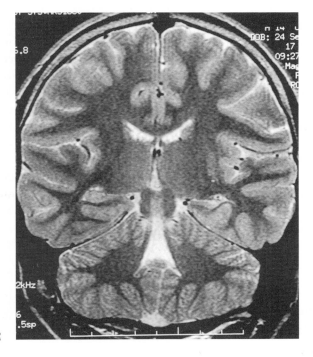

Figure 3.4
MRI: coronal view of left-sided mesial temporal (hippocampal) sclerosis.

Figure 3.5
MRI: coronal view of dysembryoplastic neuroepithelial tumour in the left temporal lobe.

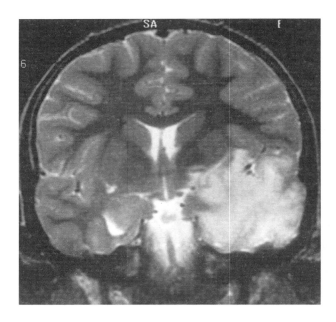

Familial temporal lobe epilepsy, usually manifesting as a familial tendency to developing *déjà vu*, is an increasingly recognized syndrome and may actually be the most common cause of familial epilepsy in adults (*see* Chapter 3).

Seizure types

The main seizure types in temporal lobe epilepsy are (alone or in combination) simple partial, complex partial and secondary generalized seizures. Seizures arise either in the amygdalo-hippocampus (e.g. in mesial temporal sclerosis) or in the lateral temporal cortex. The main functions of the temporal lobe relate to language, memory and mood, these functions being reflected in the seizure manifestations.

Simple partial seizures

These are characterized by a retention of consciousness associated with autonomic symptoms (e.g. an epigastric aura), psychic symptoms (e.g. *déjà vu*) and/or, sometimes, olfactory and auditory phenomena. Autonomic signs, including pallor or flushing, pupil dilatation, tachycardia, piloerection, sweating and cardiac arrhythmia, often accompany them:

- **Epigastric aura** is the most common, manifesting as an epigastric sensation ('butterflies') rising to the throat and mouth, sometimes with stomach pain, isolated vomiting or salivation.

- **Uncinate seizures** manifest as olfactory and gustatory symptoms (unpleasant smells or tastes) and localize to the medial temporal lobe.
- **Dysmnesic seizures** manifest as psychic symptoms and again point to a medial temporal focus. These include feelings of familiarity (*déjà vu*), unfamiliarity (*jamais vu*), memory flashbacks (often the same memory each time), depersonalization and feelings of unreality.
- **Affective seizures.** Emotional experiences such as isolated fear, laughter or rage localize to the amygdala.

Complex partial seizures

Complex partial seizures of temporal origin are characterized by:

- altered consciousness
- automatisms
- amnesia for the event.

They may be preceded by simple partial seizures, for example an epigastric aura, in about 30 per cent of cases. Typical seizures begin with motor arrest followed by oral automatism (lip smacking or grimacing). Other automatisms may include hand wringing, fiddling with clothes, walking in a circle or dressing and undressing. The episode lasts about a minute (usually 30 seconds to 3 minutes) and is followed by post-ictal confusion and amnesia.

Some information about the seizure's localization can be inferred from its characteristics (Marks and Laxer, 1998), but this is variable between individuals, is affected by the spread of the seizure discharge to neighbouring territories (especially the frontal lobe) and should be interpreted with caution:

- Staring, ictal speech, facial contractions, epigastric sensations and ictal vomiting each suggest a right-sided focus.
- *Déjà vu* and post-ictal dysphasia suggest a left-sided focus.
- Head turning to either side suggests the spread of the seizure discharge to the contralateral frontal lobe.

Secondary generalized seizures

These are the most common cause of adult-onset generalized seizures. Typical attacks begin with a simple or complex partial seizure (epigastric aura, etc.) followed by a loss of consciousness, brief limb flexion followed by extension, often with a cry (the 'tonic' phase), and then generalized repetitive limb jerking gradually replacing the tonic contraction (the 'clonic' phase). There may be incontinence, tongue biting or other self-injury. Afterwards, the patient is typically confused, disorientated, sleepy and achy, and has a headache.

Frontal lobe epilepsy

The frontal lobe is large, three times the size of the temporal lobe and comprising over a third of the brain volume. It therefore cannot be considered as a uniform whole.

Causes

Where a cause for frontal lobe epilepsy is found, it can be categorised as follows.

Lesional   Various structural lesions may lead to recurrent frontal lobe seizures. Most, for example head injury, haemorrhage or tumour, are obvious on clinical or radiological examination. Often, however, detailed radiological study with high-resolution MR scanning is needed to identify important causes of frontal lobe epilepsy such as developmental tumours (e.g. ganglioglioma and dysembryoplastic neuroepithelial tumour), cerebral dysplasia or cavernoma.

Genetic   ADNFLE is a recently recognized familial syndrome characterized by frequent, brief, sleep-related seizures starting in childhood and varying greatly in severity between members of the same family. ADNFLE is discussed elsewhere (*see* Chapter 5).

Seizure types

Supplementary motor area seizures   The supplementary motor area lies on the medial aspect of the frontal lobe, anterior to the motor cortex. Seizures arising here characteristically occur from sleep, are brief (10–40 seconds) and frequent (many per night) and show predominantly motor features, often with retained consciousness. They are of two types:

- **Frontal hyperkinetic seizures.** There is occasionally an aura on wakening from sleep (typically visceral, experiential or fear). Complex and large-amplitude seizure movements including semi-purposeful behaviour, which may lead to self-injury, follow this.
- **Postural tonic seizures.** If there is an aura, it is usually somatosensory. There then follows vocalization and asymmetric bilateral tonic posturing, sometimes including a wide-eyed grin.

Adversive seizures   Seizures arising in the frontopolar region begin with abrupt loss of consciousness followed by contraversion of the head, eyes and body. Seizures arising more posteriorly may begin with head and eye turning with retained consciousness before the convulsion.

Frontal absence seizures   This uncommon seizure arises from the fronto-polar area of the medial frontal lobe. The seizures occur typically during the daytime and begin without an aura, manifesting as speech and behaviour arrest associated with impaired consciousness for about 10–30 seconds, followed by mild post-ictal confusion.

Jacksonian seizures   These arise in the motor cortex and are the classical example of simple partial seizures. The patient may experience involuntary jerking of a finger or hand; the seizure 'marches' up the arm to the face and leg before either ending or developing into a secondary generalized convulsion.

Speech arrest   Seizures manifesting as speech arrest can be inferred to involve the speech centre in the dominant frontal lobe.

Difficulty in diagnosis

Several factors lead to difficulty in the assessment of frontal lobe seizures, and particularly confusion with non-epileptic attacks.

Supplementary motor area seizures typically are brief and occur from sleep, leading to the frequent misdiagnosis of parasomnia or just restless sleep.

Consciousness is characteristically retained during frontal lobe seizures. It is possible to have a bilateral involvement of the supplementary motor areas, and consequent bilateral tonic-clonic limb activity, without involvement of the remainder of the cortex, thus consciousness being retained. This situation had traditionally previously been regarded as a feature of non-epileptic attacks.

Hyperventilation is a characteristic feature of supplementary motor seizures. This, together with the increase in seizure frequency at times of anxiety, may lead to an erroneous diagnosis of psychogenic non-epileptic attack disorder.

Seizures confined to the supplementary motor area are buried between the cerebral hemispheres so may be undetectable on surface EEG (the ictal EEG may show only movement artefact).

The two frontal lobes have close connections via the corpus callosum such that unilateral frontal seizures can rapidly become bilateral or generalize. Such generalized seizures occurring without aura and sometimes with apparently simultaneously bilateral EEG changes are easily misdiagnosed as primarily generalized seizures.

Intimate connections between the frontal and temporal lobes may sometimes mean that seizures arising in the frontal lobe manifest as temporal lobe seizures. Many cryptogenic localization-related epilepsies originally considered to be of temporal lobe origin are now recognized to arise in the frontal lobes.

Table 3.2
Characteristics of frontal
seizures that distinguish
them from temporal lobe
seizures

- Seizures most commonly occur from sleep
- Seizures are very frequent (e.g. daily or many times per night) and often clustered
- Attacks are brief (10–30 seconds)
- Some consciousness may be retained despite generalized movements
- Motor features, e.g. postural changes, excessive limb movements, purposeless activity or non-directed violence with self-injury (frontal hyperkinetic seizures) are prominent
- Vocalizations including shouting or loud groaning are common
- There may be 'absences' manifesting as arrest of speech and/or behaviour with impaired consciousness
- Post-ictal confusion is brief or absent
- The EEG is often normal between episodes and may even be normal during attacks
- There is a high rate of spontaneous remission

The main features that distinguish frontal from temporal lobe seizures are listed in Table 3.2.

Parietal lobe epilepsy

This uncommon epilepsy usually presents with sensory symptoms, either tingling or pain (Sveinbjornsdottir and Duncan, 1993), which begin in one area and 'march' in a way similar to the Jacksonian frontal seizure. Disorders of higher spatial function (apraxia and anosognosia) may accompany the seizures. Sexual seizures are a rare manifestation of epilepsy involving the parietal paracentral lobule.

Occipital lobe epilepsy

The seizure semiology of occipital epilepsy is identical whether the cause is symptomatic, for example from a tumour, or idiopathic, such as from late-onset benign occipital epilepsy. (The seizures of early-onset benign occipital epilepsy are described elsewhere.)

Visual seizures are brief and frequent, and may manifest as any visual symptom from blurred vision, lights (phosphenes) and illusions to hallucinations (see Plate 1), palinopsia (persistent images) and visual blackening.

Patients are almost always aware that the images are not real. Zigzags are rare and usually imply migraine. Vertiginous seizures, eye turning (usually towards the side of the focus), eyelid flutter or rapid blinking may occur.

The EEG may show lateralized abnormalities; the main difference between symptomatic and late-onset benign occipital epilepsy is the failure of the EEG in symptomatic forms to respond to eye opening or closing.

Causes of symptomatic epilepsy

The major causes of symptomatic epilepsy are listed below:

- mesial temporal (hippocampal) sclerosis
- malformations of cerebral development
- tumours
- cerebrovascular disorders
- injury
- infection and inflammation
- biochemical and metabolic.

Mesial temporal sclerosis

Mesial temporal lobe epilepsy is the best characterized adult-onset, localization-related epilepsy. It may commence in childhood. The pathological substrate for the condition is mesial temporal sclerosis, or scarring in the hippocampal formations of the medial temporal lobe (*see* Fig. 3.4). The clinical recognition of mesial temporal lobe epilepsy is important as it is potentially curable with surgery. Several characteristics, described below, allow it to be considered as an epilepsy syndrome.

An **early life event**, characteristically before the age of 4 years, is crucial to the expression of the disorder. Examples might include infection, trauma or febrile seizure (particularly if prolonged and lateralized). It is likely that mesial temporal (hippocampal) sclerosis develops at this stage in the developing and vulnerable brain. An increased prevalence of neuronal migration abnormalities suggests a pre-existing vulnerability to developing mesial temporal sclerosis. It is also possible that the subsequent frequent seizures themselves are important in the genesis of mesial temporal sclerosis.

A **latent interval** follows before epilepsy develops; this may vary from a few weeks to many years.

Temporal lobe **seizures** associated with mesial temporal sclerosis have several consistent features:

- an epigastric aura, often in isolation, in 80 per cent of cases
- predominantly complex partial nature with rare tonic-clonic seizures
- relative resistance to medication.

The **EEG** shows anterior temporal spikes between seizures; these are bilateral and independent in 50 per cent, although predominating on the affected side. EEG during a seizure shows lateralized theta to alpha rhythms, which are over the affected side in up to 95 per cent of cases.

MRI is essential in the evaluation of temporal lobe epilepsy; coronal views through the hippocampal region show hippocampal atrophy, often with mesial temporal sclerosis (*see* Fig 3.4 above). 'Inversion recovery' MRI sequences give the best grey matter/white matter differential, so this is the preferred method of hippocampal imaging. The difference in size between the right and left hippocampi is a more reliable indication of hippocampal sclerosis than is the signal change (which is not always present). The size difference is best appreciated in the body of the hippocampus rather than the tail or head.

An associated feature of hippocampal sclerosis is an ipsilateral reduction in the size of the temporal lobe and of the fornix. Dual pathology is also surprisingly common. For example, 25 per cent of cases of cortical dysplasia and 2 per cent of low-grade gliomas presenting with epilepsy have associated hippocampal sclerosis.

Functional imaging, for example positron emission tomography (PET) scanning, shows hypometabolism in the affected temporal lobe but may show more widespread evidence of dysfunction than is apparent on MRI.

On **surgery**, the finding of ipsilateral hippocampal atrophy correlates with success of surgery in controlling seizures.

Pathology of the resected hippocampus shows pyramidal cell loss in hippocampal zones CA1 and CA3 with mesial temporal sclerosis; surprisingly, the pathological changes are bilateral in up to 80 per cent of cases.

Malformations of cerebral (particularly cortical) development

Malformations of the cerebral cortex are increasingly recognized as a cause of learning disability and epilepsy (Walsh, 1999). The disorders represent a heterogeneous group with a wide spectrum of clinical presentation and differing underlying causes, pathology and imaging features. They are epileptogenic to varying degrees. Overall, congenital cortical abnormalities are found in about 5 per cent of adults and 15 per cent of children with epilepsy, particularly those with learning disabilities. Other cerebral malformations are less likely to predispose to epilepsy.

Normal brain development

When considering how alterations in cerebral formation might predispose to epilepsy, an understanding of normal development is helpful.

Neurulation   Neuralation with the formation of the neural tube from ectoderm occurs from 4–6 weeks' gestation. There is a rapid multiplication of neuronal cells in the periventricular region at this time, and up to about 10 weeks' gestation.

Migration   The migration of neuronal cells from the periventricular regions to the cortical areas occurs between 4 and 24 weeks' gestation, the maximal migration occurring at between 10 and 20 weeks. Migration is mainly radial, the cells forming the inner cortical layers migrating first, and those migrating later moving beyond the inner layers to increasingly more peripheral positions. Once in the cortex, neurones may migrate laterally, particularly if they are destined to form part of the ventrolateral and lateral parts of the anterior cortex. Considering the complexity of migration, relatively frequent aberrations are to be expected.

Organization   The organization of interneuronal connections occurs maximally as migration is completed, from about 20 weeks' gestation to 6–12 months of postnatal life. Dendritic and axonal outgrowth is associated with the release of neurotransmitters. Synapse formation is a relatively late event. Initially, there is an overproduction of synapses, so that the maximal number is present at about 6–12 months postnatally, with a subsequent selective pruning and an associated loss of some neurones. The number of synapses remains high until 2–3 years but reduces to an adult level between 5 and 10 years.

The establishment and elimination of synapses are clearly important in the context of epilepsy. Seizure discharges may reinforce unwanted or aberrant synaptic connections, to the detriment of establishing more desirable pathways.

Abnormal brain development (as a cause of epilepsy)

These conditions may be classified according to the stage of brain development (Barkovich *et al.*, 1996).

Abnormal glial and neuronal proliferation

Conditions associated with foci of abnormal cellular proliferation include neurocutaneous syndromes (e.g. tuberous sclerosis) and hamartomatous benign tumours (e.g. ganglioglioma or dysembryoplastic neuroepithelial tumour [DNET]).

Tuberous sclerosis (epiloia) is an uncommon (1 in 30 000) but important cause of childhood-onset epilepsy and learning disability. Two separate genotypes at chromosomes 9q.34 (*TFC*1) and l6p.l3 (*TFC*2) code for the tumour suppressor proteins hamartin and tuberin respectively.

The manifestations of tuberous sclerosis are highly variable, involving mainly the nervous system and skin. Seizures occur in 80 per cent of cases, usually from the first year of life. Tuberous sclerosis is an important cause of

West syndrome: it should be considered in all who present with infantile spasms. Learning disability is found in 50 per cent of cases, almost all of which have early-onset seizures. Brain hamartomas (tubers) are seen as calcified subependymal nodules on cerebral imaging in the majority. Histologically, these show characteristic balloon cells. Malignant brain tumours occasionally develop (subependymal giant cell astrocytomas).

There are four characteristic skin lesions:

- **Adenoma sebaceum** are skin hamartomas (angiokeratomas) over the nose and cheeks. These are not seen in young children.
- **Periungual fibromata** occur in the nail folds and beneath the nails of the hands and feet. They are also unusual in children.
- **Shagreen patch** is a fibrous plaque, usually over the lumbar region.
- **Depigmentation** in the shape of a mountain ash leaf may be visible in ordinary light but is better seen using an ultraviolet (Wood's) light. This is usually the only manifestation in infants and young children. If the scalp is affected, patches of white hair occur.

Renal involvement occurs in 60 per cent of cases, including angiomyolipomas in 50 per cent and simple renal cysts in 30 per cent. Cysts also occur in the liver and spleen. Cardiac rhabdomyomas are most likely to be found in young infants and may regress spontaneously.

Other hamartomatous lesions are considered with tumours below.

Abnormal neuronal migration

This group comprises the majority of the cortical maldevelopment syndromes:

- **Generalized** migration disorders include lissencephaly, subcortical band heterotopia and Aicardi syndrome.
- **Focal** disorders include nodular heterotopias, focal pachygyria and hemimegencephaly.

'**Lissencephaly**' literally means 'smooth brain'. Pathologically, there is loss of the brain's normal gyri and sulci (Fig. 3.6). Lissencephaly occurs in a group of conditions that are clinically, genetically, radiologically and histologically heterogeneous. One severe form is pachygyria ('pachy' thick), referring to a brain in which an abnormally thick cortex impedes normal gyration, leading to a brain with a small surface area and few or no gyri.

Classical (type I) lissencephaly is always associated with severe mental retardation, feeding problems and intractable epilepsy (frequently including infantile spasms). It occurs in three main circumstances:

- **Isolated lissencephaly sequence** is not associated with any other major anomaly. The gene associated with isolated lissencephaly sequence further defines

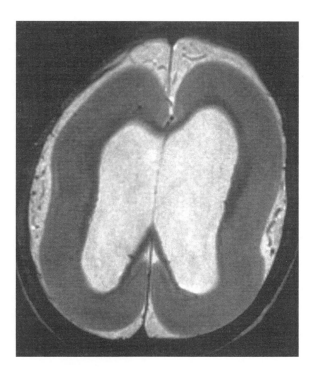

Figure 3.6
MRI:
agyria/lissencephaly.

the condition. ILS17 is associated with deletions or mutations of the *LIS-1* gene on chromosome 17p13.3. Locations for genes other than those on chromosome 17 are under investigation in isolated lissencephaly sequence.

- **X-linked lissencephaly** causes classical lissencephaly in heterozygous males and subcortical band heterotopia in carrier females. The gene responsible for this condition lies between Xq21.3 and Xq21.4. Subcortical band heterotopia, otherwise known as double cortex, occurs as a result of normal neuronal migration by neurones with normal X chromosomes and arrested migration by those carrying the X-linked lissencephaly gene.
- **Lissencephaly can occur with other malformations,** as in the Miller–Dieker syndrome and Baraitser–Winter syndrome. In Miller–Dieker syndrome, deletions of neighbouring genes, in addition to *LIS-1*, contribute to the phenotype. The gene for a syndrome of lissencephaly with cerebellar hypoplasia has not been located.

Cobblestone (type II) lissencephalies are associated with muscle and eye disease, as in Fukuyama congenital muscular dystrophy. Patients are less likely to present with seizures than those with classical lissencephaly.

Aicardi syndrome occurs only in females. The gene location is thought to be at Xp22.3. Severe mental retardation, infantile spasms, choroido-retinal lacunae and agenesis of the corpus callosum are seen clinically. Pathologically, the cortex is thin and unlayered, there is diffuse unlayered polymicrogyria, and heterotopic nodules are found in the periventricular region and the hemispheric white matter.

In **nodular heterotopias**, there is a failure of normal migration of some neurones, which results in their accumulation in abnormal positions in the white matter. X-linked subcortical band heterotopias have already been considered.

With **focal nodular heterotopias**, although the heterotopias may occur anywhere along the migration pathway, they are usually found around the ventricles and are referred to as periventricular nodular heterotopias (Fig. 3.7). They are visible on MRI, projecting from the ventricular walls into the ventricles, giving an appearance similar to that of tuberous sclerosis.

Bilateral symmetrical periventricular nodular heterotopias occur almost exclusively in females. The gene has been mapped to Xq28. This defect was considered lethal for males, but some males with this condition, cerebellar hypoplasia, severe retardation, epilepsy and syndactyly, as well as others with additional congenital malformations, have been described. Disability in females with bilateral symmetrical periventricular nodular heterotopias is

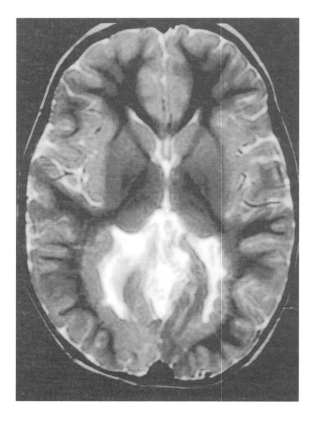

Figure 3.7
MRI: periventricular heterotopic nodules of grey matter.

very variable. Some patients start to have epilepsy early and have serious cognitive problems; others are of normal or near-normal intelligence with an onset of mild seizure disorders in late childhood or adolescence. The male offspring of affected females linked to Xp28 are normal.

Focal pachygyria exists when the gyri are reduced in number but not completely absent. Cell migration has progressed to a later stage than in lissencephaly.

Hemimegalencephaly is a hamartomatous overgrowth of all or part of one cerebral hemisphere. The neurones are abnormal, and their migration and organization are aberrant. An intractable seizure disorder starts early in life, with an accompanying contralateral hemiplegia and learning difficulties. Hemimegalencephaly can be associated with neurocutaneous syndromes, such as the epidermal nevus syndrome, unilateral hypomelanosis of Ito and neurofibromatosis type 1. Neuro-imaging shows that the hemisphere is abnormal from the ventricular wall to the cortex, the latter usually being thickened with broad gyri shallow sulci and irregularities at the grey–white matter junction. The ipsilateral lateral ventricle is enlarged.

Abnormal cortical organization

Here, damage follows the arrival of neurones at the cortex. Such conditions include polymicrogyria and schizencephaly.

In these conditions, the area from which seizures arise (the epileptogenic zone) may be adjacent to, not necessarily within, the area of visible abnormality on cerebral imaging; functional imaging is therefore essential before undertaking epilepsy surgery for these conditions.

In **polymicrogyria**, the neurones reach the cortex but are abnormally distributed. The cortical gyri are narrow and have an abnormal convolutional pattern (Plate 3). In unlayered microgyria, a single cell layer undulates between the white matter and the molecular layer – there are often co-existing anomalies such as agenesis of the corpus callosum. In classical four-layer microgyria, the histological appearance suggests that adverse events have occurred after migration, towards the fifth and sixth months of gestation. Insults leading to reduced perfusion of the fetal brain, with resultant hypoxia, are thought to be responsible.

The clinical presentation can be very variable. The severity of mental retardation, neurological handicap and epilepsy relates to the extent of the cortical involvement. On neuro-imaging, polymicrogyria is isodense to normal cortex, calcification is seen in a small proportion of cases, and anomalous venous drainage is common.

Congenital bilateral perisylvian syndrome consists of oropharyngeal dysfunction, leading to severe feeding difficulties, dysarthria, epilepsy, mental retardation and occasionally arthrogryposis. Neuro-imaging shows bilateral central rolandic and sylvian macrogyria with thickened cortex. The macrogyria are shown pathologically to be collections of microgyria.

Unilateral opercular dysplasia may be associated with relatively benign forms of epilepsy.

The anomaly **schizencephaly** is a grey matter-lined cleft spanning the cerebral hemisphere to the lateral ventricle. The cleft may be open or closed, unilateral or bilateral. Epilepsy and various degrees of motor and mental handicap occur. It is thought that schizencephaly results from an ischaemic injury to the developing cortex soon after the migrational stage. However, the recent finding of germ line mutations of the homeobox gene *EMX2* in patients with schizencephaly suggests that genetic factors can be important.

Tumours

Tumours are a major cause of epilepsy in adults. In general, tumours that present with epilepsy are more slowly growing and have a better overall prognosis. Epilepsy from certain low-grade tumours (*see* below) may be very resistant to medical treatment; epilepsy from more malignant tumours is often easier to control, but clearly the tumour itself is more serious.

Benign tumours

Some relatively benign tumours are visible only on MR scanning, making this an essential investigation in patients with focal epilepsy, especially if the seizures are difficult to control.

Dysembryoplastic neuroepithelial tumour (DNET) is a hamartomatous lesion rather than a neoplasm. Although rare, it comprises 12 per cent of brain tumours that require surgery for resistant epilepsy. It is usually located in the temporal lobe (*see* Fig. 3.5 above). It presents with young-onset, refractory partial seizures without neurological or intellectual deficit. The lesion remains unchanged over time. Characteristically, it is a multinodular intracortical lesion that appears cystic on MRI. Histologically, it comprises three cell types: oligodendroglia, astrocytes and infrequent ganglion cells.

Gangliogliomas are slow growing, usually of childhood onset and almost always lead to treatment-resistant epilepsy. Although rare (1 per cent of all brain tumours), they represent some 50 per cent of brain tumours that come to surgery for resistant epilepsy. They are frequently overlooked, such that 10 years from seizure onset until surgery for ganglioglioma is usual.

On MRI (essential for its diagnosis), a ganglioglioma appears as a discrete cortical lesion (high signal on T2, low on T1), usually with a central cystic area. Histologically it has, as its name suggests, two components: ganglion cells (malformed heterotopic neurones) and glial cells (astrocytes). It is the glial component that grows; the ganglion cells are maladaptive but not neoplastic. As with other cortical development abnormalities, there are often clusters of similar cells in the neighbouring brain that may be missed on MRI.

Meningioma commonly causes adult-onset seizures.

With a **hypothalamic hamartoma**, symptoms start towards the end of the first decade. The seizures are characterized by uncontrollable laughter (gelastic seizures), and there may be secondary generalized attacks later. Deterioration in cognitive function, striking and intractable aggression, hyperactivity and poor judgement are usual but not invariable.

Malignant tumours

Low-grade astrocytomas and **oligodendrogliomas** are the most common tumours leading to intractable epilepsy. Those presenting with epilepsy usually arise in the temporal lobe and have a much better prognosis than those presenting without epilepsy. Such tumours usually have a long history of seizures before surgery (mean 7–15 years) and favourable biological behaviour following surgery.

High-grade astrocytoma (glioblastoma multiforme) presents surprisingly rarely with epilepsy.

Giant cell astrocytoma is the glioma found typically in tuberous sclerosis. It arises in the subependymal areas. The large, bizarre cells have the appearance of atypical astrocytes: they are often multinucleated and vacuolated. The tumours typically arise in the vicinity of the caudate nucleus, often leading to obstruction of the foramen of Monro. A deterioration in seizure control in tuberous sclerosis is often the indicator of a developing giant cell astrocytoma.

Metastatic brain tumours frequently present as epilepsy, especially when involving the cerebral cortex.

Cerebrovascular disorders

Cerebrovascular disease is a common cause of epilepsy in adults. It accounts for much of the steeply rising incidence of epilepsy in the elderly.

Stroke

Stroke, either ischaemic or haemorrhagic, affecting the cerebral cortex (but not deep lacunar lesions) is a common cause of epilepsy. The risk of seizures in the first 2 weeks after an acute stroke is about 5 per cent (Kilpatrick *et al.*, 1990). Overall, the risk of seizures in the first 5 years following a stroke is 11.5 per cent (Burn *et al.*, 1997). The risk is highest for large strokes and haemorrhagic lesions, and in the elderly. Venous infarctions in the cortex are particularly epileptogenic.

Arteriovenous malformation

Overall, about 20 per cent of arteriovenous malformations present with epilepsy, most of the remainder presenting with haemorrhage (Crawford *et al.*, 1986). Those presenting as epilepsy tended to be larger and more superficial. Conventional arteriovenous malformation surgery reduces the haemorrhage risk but greatly increases the risk of subsequent epilepsy. Other treatment approaches include stereotactic radiotherapy and embolization.

Cavernous angioma (cavernoma)

Although cavernomas are uncommon, epilepsy is a frequent complication, particularly when they involve the cortex. Some cases are familial. About half of cavernomas found on cerebral imaging have presented with epilepsy. Obvious haemorrhage is rare (approximately 0.7 per cent per year [Robinson *et al.*, 1991]), but very minor bleeding causing haemosiderin deposition around the lesion is usual; this is probably the irritant that causes the seizures. Also, neuronal dysplasia sometimes lies adjacent to the lesion. Surgery for cavernoma includes the removal of some surrounding brain tissue to ensure that the epileptogenic zone is removed.

Others

Vasculitis of the nervous system, either primary (isolated cranial angiitis) or secondary to systemic vasculitis, infection or lymphoma, may present with seizures as well as headache and localizing signs. The encephalopathy of hypertension and eclampsia is particularly likely to cause seizures. Cerebral hypoperfusion following cardiac arrest is often associated with post-anoxic myoclonus and seizures. Surgery for congenital cardiac disorders carries a small but definite risk of stroke and associated epilepsy.

Head injury

The risk of developing seizures is increased following significant head trauma, particularly so following penetrating injuries or intracranial bleeding. Iron deposits and haemosiderin within the brain are potently epileptogenic, perhaps increasingly so with the passage of time. This is a major factor leading to post-traumatic epilepsy. It is difficult to quantify precisely the risk following a head injury since all the larger studies have been retrospective. Minor head trauma and epilepsy are both common conditions; many people with epilepsy can recall previous minor head injuries, but these are rarely relevant to their seizures.

Timing of seizures after injury

Epilepsy following head injury is broadly divided into three types, depending upon the time since the injury:

1. **Immediate (concussive) seizures.** 'Concussive' convulsions occur within seconds of an acute head injury. Memorable examples of this are seen in videos of Australian Rules footballers (McCrory *et al.*, 1997). These events are not considered to be epileptic, are not associated with typical EEG changes and do not predict the later occurrence of epilepsy.

2. **Early (traumatic) seizures.** Seizures occurring within a week (and commonly within an hour) of trauma are likely in young children. Although 75 per cent have no further seizures after the first week, 25 per cent will go on to develop late (post-traumatic) epilepsy.

3. **Late (post-traumatic) epilepsy.** Seizures occurring more than 1 week after head trauma imply a long-term seizure tendency. Seizures develop within a year in about half of cases and within 4 years in a further 25 per cent; seizures relating to the injury may occasionally occur as long as 40 years later. Post-traumatic epilepsy is often difficult to control on medication.

Site of post-traumatic seizure onset

Frontal and temporal lobe epilepsies are the most common forms following closed head injury. This is because the frontal and temporal regions are the major sites of brain injury (contusion or intracerebral bleeding) following closed head trauma, irrespective of the direction and site of the impact. The brain is thrown forwards against the anterior walls of the frontal and middle cerebral fossae, and the delicate undersurface of the brain is rubbed against the rough skull base, causing contusion and haemorrhage (Fig. 3.8).

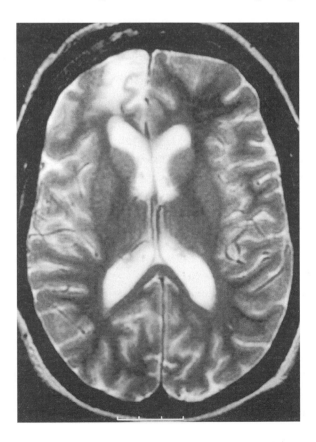

Figure 3.8
MRI: axial view of a (previous) head injury with right frontal contusion.

Table 3.3
The standardized incidence (compared with the non-injured population) of developing post-traumatic epilepsy at various times following injuries of varying severity (data from Annegers *et al.*, 1998)

Injury type	< 1 year	1–9 years	> 10 years
Mild	3	1.5	1
Moderate	7	3	2
Severe	95	15	4
Penetrating (war)	580	25	–

Risk of developing post-traumatic epilepsy

There is a strong relationship between the severity of traumatic brain injury and the subsequent risk of developing post-traumatic epilepsy. The severity of a head injury can be broadly divided into three categories:

- **Mild.** There is loss of consciousness or post-traumatic amnesia lasting less than 30 minutes, with no skull fracture.
- **Moderate.** There is either loss of consciousness or post-traumatic amnesia of between 30 minutes and 24 hours, or a skull fracture.
- **Severe.** There is either brain contusion or intracerebral haematoma, or a loss of consciousness or post-traumatic amnesia of more than 24 hours. The highest risk of epilepsy from head trauma is from penetrating (missile) injuries, such as those seen during warfare.

The standardized incidence (compared with the non-injured population) of developing post-traumatic epilepsy following an injury of each severity is given in Table 3.3. The risk is clearly highest in the first year, but following severe injuries, some risk persists for decades.

The cumulative probability of an individual developing post-traumatic epilepsy is as follows (Annegers *et al.*, 1998):

- Mild injury: 0.7 per cent at 5 years, 2 per cent at 30 years.
- Moderate injury: 1.2 per cent at 5 years, 4 per cent at 30 years.
- Severe injury: 10 per cent at 5 years, 17 per cent at 30 years.

Table 3.4 lists the factors influencing the chance of a head injury leading to epilepsy.

Role of prophylactic anti-epileptic medication following head injury

Seizures occurring in the acute stage following a severe head injury may damage an already vulnerable brain by worsening hypoxia, increasing metabolic demand and causing excess neurotransmitter release. Besides preventing

Factors favouring the development of post-traumatic epilepsy	Factors unrelated to the development of post-traumatic epilepsy
Brain contusion with intracerebral haemorrhage. The risk may be as high as 35% following surgery for acute traumatic intracranial haematoma	The **EEG**, perhaps surprisingly, does not help in predicting the likelihood of late seizures
Skull fracture. The risk may be as high as 20% following depressed skull vault fractures, especially if the fracture is accompanied by prolonged post-traumatic amnesia, penetration of the dura or focal neurological signs	A positive **family history** of epilepsy appears not to influence the risk
Early (traumatic) epilepsy is a marker of injury severity and is associated with a 25% risk of developing post-traumatic epilepsy	Prophylactic **anti-epileptic medication** can suppress seizures but does not influence the underlying tendency to develop epilepsy (see text)
Loss of consciousness or post-traumatic amnesia for more than 24 hours	
Age over 65 years	

Table 3.4

Pointers predicting the outcome in relation to epilepsy following head injury

acute seizures, some anti-epileptic medications may, in theory, be neuro-protective by blocking sodium channels and thus reducing excitotoxic neuro-transmitter release. Conversely, the toxicity of anti-epileptic medication may, in theory, be greater in the acutely injured brain. Unfortunately, anti-epileptic medication does not seem to prevent death or disability from acute head trauma.

The limited role for prophylactic anti-epileptic medication is as follows (Schierhout and Roberts, 1998):

- Anti-epileptic medication, for example phenytoin, can be recommended for the acute stage of brain injury (e.g. the first 2 weeks after severe head trauma), since it suppresses the tendency towards early seizures.
- Anti-epileptic medication does not prevent the development of a late seizure tendency and so need not be continued beyond 2 weeks unless late

Table 3.5
Factors suggesting that an individual's epilepsy can be attributed to head injury

- There was no history of seizures prior to the head injury
- The head injury was moderate or severe
- There was a penetrating injury or depressed skull fracture
- There was an intracranial haematoma
- The onset of seizures following head trauma was short (less than 1 year)
- The seizures are partial (either frontal or temporal)
- There is evidence of structural brain injury on cerebral imaging
- The clinical or EEG seizure characteristics coincide with the site of brain injury on imaging
- The EEG shows no evidence of generalized seizure activity or photosensitivity
- There are no other disorders that might cause epilepsy
- There is no family history of epilepsy

epilepsy develops, i.e. unless two or more unprovoked seizures occur 1 week or more after the injury.

Features suggesting a traumatic cause

Table 3.5 lists the main factors that help to decide whether a head injury has caused a person's epilepsy.

Infection and inflammation

Epilepsy can be associated with acute or chronic infection, related to the pathological consequences of infection and/or to alterations in cerebral function secondary to infection, but not directly to the organisms themselves. Bacterial, viral, protozoal, fungal and parasitic infections can all be involved.

Meningitis

- **Viral.** With the exception of seizures as a non-specific response to fever in young children, epileptic attacks are uncommon in viral meningitis.
- **Bacterial.** Pure inflammation of the meninges is not usually associated with acute or chronic seizures. However, underlying cerebritis, or the development of associated vasculitis with secondary cerebral ischaemia

(particularly prominent in tuberculous meningitis), may cause cortical irritation and seizures during the acute phase.

Encephalitis

Seizures are a common feature of acute encephalitis. Herpes simplex encephalitis is particularly liable to present with persisting focal attacks, but any other encephalitic illnesses may be complicated by seizures. In tropical countries, cerebral malaria is an important cause in childhood. A high proportion of those whose encephalitic illness is complicated by seizures will have continuing epilepsy later.

Prenatal infections with organisms such as *Toxoplasma* and cytomegalovirus lead to cerebral scarring, with epilepsy as a consequence of earlier infection. Infection with herpes hominis virus types 6 and 7 is considered to be a precursor of mesial temporal sclerosis in some patients. The encephalopathy of HIV infection is not itself associated with seizures, but the immunodeficiency allows infection with opportunist organisms such as cytomegalovirus, which may be more epileptogenic. Similarly, children who have been treated with cranial radiotherapy or chemotherapy for malignant disease are at risk of viral encephalitic illnesses, which can predispose to epilepsy.

Cysticercosis

Cysticerosis, derived from poor sanitation and eating undercooked pork, is one of the most frequent causes of epilepsy worldwide, especially in Latin America (Garcia *et al.*, 1993). Scattered calcifications in the brain parenchyma are apparent on CT scanning.

Rasmussen's encephalitis

This condition manifests as intractable seizures (especially simple partial seizures) associated with progressive cortical atrophy and patchy inflammation. It is usually of childhood onset. An autoimmune aetiology due to an underlying viral infection (e.g. cytomegalovirus) is suspected; the finding of occasional antibodies to anti-glutamate receptor subunit 3 supports this hypothesis.

Biochemical and metabolic causes

Epilepsy may, particularly in young children, be associated with the direct or indirect effects of metabolic derangement.

Direct effects

- **Glucose:** low blood glucose level; low cerebrospinal fluid glucose with normal blood glucose in glucose transporter deficiency.
- **Pyridoxine (vitamin B6)** dependency usually presents in the neonatal period, but later onset has been recorded.
- **GABA transaminase** deficiency is associated with somatic overgrowth and spongiform degeneration of the myelin.
- **Ammonia.** A high level usually results from a deficiency of enzymes in the urea cycle. Patients present neonatally, but the onset may be later if the deficiency is incomplete.
- **Glycine.** Non-ketotic hyperglycinaemia is one of the causes of early myoclonic encephalopathy.
- **Glutaric acid.** Acute-onset seizures are associated with dystonia in glutaric aciduria type 1.

Indirect effects

- **Peroxisomal disorders** such as Zellweger syndrome, pseudo-Zellweger syndrome and neonatal adrenoleukodystrophy are associated with cortical dysplasia.
- **Sulphite oxidase and molybdenum co-factor deficiencies** lead to severe cerebral damage, with therapy-resistant seizures.

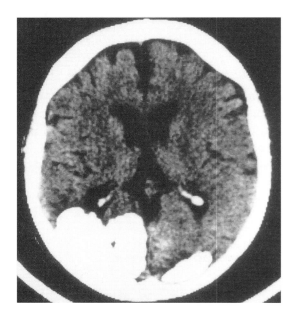

Figure 3.9
Computed tomography brain scan: occipital calcifications in coeliac disease presenting as an adult with occipital epilepsy.

- **Biotinidase deficiency** leads to lactic acidaemia with seizures, extreme hypotonia, *Candida* skin infections and alopecia.
- **Mitochondrial dysfunction.** MELAS (mitochondrial myopathy, encephalopathy, lactic acidosis, and stroke-like episodes) and MERRF (*see* Plate 2) are the most clearly defined mitochondrial disorders, but seizures also occur in less well-characterized disorders of mitochondrial function.
- **Coeliac disease.** This may cause a variety of nervous system manifestations including epilepsy. The seizures typically arise in the occipital lobe and are associated with intracerebral calcification (Fig. 3.9).

The differential diagnosis of epilepsy

Introduction

The differential diagnosis of altered consciousness, with or without associated movement, is very broad. The most common disorders confused with seizures are syncope and psychogenic attacks (anxiety, hyperventilation and non-epileptic convulsions) and, in children, breath-holding spells and reflex anoxic attacks. Even within these groups, there are many different conditions, requiring a different approach to treatment. Table 4.1 lists some common reasons for a misdiagnosis of epilepsy.

Syncope

Syncope is a complicated problem frequently encountered in clinical practice. The majority of adults presenting to a 'first seizure' clinic have syncope. Syncope describes a loss of consciousness, usually from a sudden decrease in cerebral blood flow (*synkoptein*, Greek = 'to cut off'). The brain can withstand only a few seconds of total interruption of blood flow without loss of

Table 4.1
Common problems in diagnosing episodes of altered consciousness

- The history is often inadequate if the attack was unwitnessed or a witness is unavailable

- A history of clonic movements or incontinence in syncope or non-epileptic attacks may lead to an erroneous diagnosis of epilepsy

- Undeserved emphasis may be placed upon 'abnormal' EEG findings, e.g. when these may be normal or age-specific variants

- A family history of epilepsy or a history of febrile convulsions does not necessarily favour a diagnosis of epilepsy

Table 4.2
The clinical distinction of syncope from seizures (*indicating the most important distinguishing features)

	Seizure	Syncope
Trigger*	Rare (flashing lights, hyperventilation)	Common (upright position, bathroom, blood, needles, exertion)
Prodrome	Common (typical aura: epigastric, *déjà vu*, etc.)	Almost always (nausea, sweating, palpitation, light-headedness, visual darkening)
Onset	May be sudden	Gradual (often minutes)
Duration	1–2 minutes	1–30 seconds
Convulsive jerks	Common (prolonged)	Common (brief)
Incontinence	Common	Uncommon
Lateral tongue bite*	Common	Rare
Colour	Pale (simple partial seizure) Red, blue (tonic–clonic seizure)	Very pale
Post-ictal recovery	Slow (confused)	Rapid (quickly orientated)
Post-ictal confusion*	Common (e.g. wakes in the ambulance)	Rare (e.g. wakes on the floor)

consciousness. The distinction of syncope from epilepsy is very important (Table 4.2) and relies upon a detailed history and witness account.

Syncope is classified according to its probable cause. Most syncope can be classified either as reflex (vasovagal) or orthostatic; less common but often more serious causes include cardiac, respiratory and central nervous system syncope.

REFLEX (VASOVAGAL) SYNCOPE

This is the most common form, affecting mainly children and young adults. It is caused by an exaggeration of normal cardiovascular reflexes and so is seen in otherwise healthy individuals with an intact autonomic response. It therefore differs from orthostatic syncope, which is associated with a failing autonomic response.

Clinical features

Triggers

There are usually precipitating factors such as prolonged standing, rising from lying or emotional trauma, including pain, venepuncture or the sight of blood. Vasovagal syncope typically occurs in the bathroom, in the doctor's surgery or in hot, crowded areas.

Prodrome

The onset is gradual, with pre-syncopal symptoms of light-headedness, nausea, sweating, palpitation, greying or blacking of the vision, a muffling of hearing, a feeling of being distant from the surroundings, etc.

The blackout

There is typically pallor, sweating and cold skin. The muscle tone is flaccid and there may be a few uncoordinated clonic jerks, but these do not precede the fall. Movement and jerking during a blackout are quite consistent with syncope (Lempert *et al.*, 1994). A common error is to label syncope as a seizure based upon a witness account of shaking. Incontinence and injury are uncommon and lateral tongue biting rare. Recovery is usually rapid with no confusion.

Investigations

The history often leaves little doubt about the syncopal nature of the attacks, with further investigation not being required. Investigations sometimes indicated include the following:

- **Blood pressure** may fall from lying to standing, together with a rise in pulse rate; in practice, this test is poorly sensitive for vasovagal syncope.
- **Blood tests** will exclude anaemia and hyponatraemia.
- An **ECG** will detect arrhythmias, including Wolff–Parkinson–White syndrome, long QT syndrome (*see* below), etc.
- **Tilt table testing** (60° tilt for 45 minutes) is an important investigation, highly sensitive (up to 90 per cent) and specific (70 per cent) for a syncopal tendency. Measures to induce syncope, for example isoprenaline, may provoke more rapid syncope, but the resulting lowered specificity argues against its usefulness.

Management

An explanation of the problem and advice on posture – head down or lie flat at symptom onset, or rise slowly from lying – are often sufficient. Behavioural psychotherapy including systematic desensitization, for example to the sight of blood, is often successful where there are specific triggers. Beta-blockers or selective serotonin reuptake inhibitors are sometimes used. A cardiac pacemaker may be indicated for severe (malignant) vasovagal syncope or for the related condition of carotid sinus hypersensitivity.

CAROTID SINUS SYNCOPE

Carotid sinus hypersensitivity is identified in up to 20 per cent of people over 60 years of age, particularly men. About 20 per cent of cases present with syncope attributable to carotid pressure, for example from a tight collar or head turning.

Carotid sinus massage must be performed only under ECG and blood pressure monitoring, and with the patient supine. Each carotid artery is massaged separately for 5–15 seconds (leaving at least 15 seconds between sides). A positive response is cardio-inhibitory (a sinus pause of > 3 seconds) or vasodepressive (a blood pressure fall of > 50 mmHg), or mixed.

The risks of massage include prolonged asystole, transient or permanent neurological deficit and sudden death. Massage should be avoided if there is obvious cerebrovascular disease.

REFLEX ANOXIC ATTACKS

These cause diagnostic confusion in young children. They result from brief asystole due to excessive vagus nerve activity. Sudden unexpected events that may involve pain are the most likely precipitants.

The blackout

There is immediate loss of consciousness and tone, elevation of the eyes, and extreme pallor with a dusky colour to the lips. Seconds later, stiffening in extension, with fisting of the hands, clenching of the jaw and a few clonic jerks are seen. Within 30 seconds, relaxation with a somewhat far-away expression is followed by a brief period of crying and the child sleeps for a while. Attacks can be very frequent.

Diagnosis

This is almost invariably made on the history, but, if necessary, can be confirmed by inducing an attack. Bilateral ocular pressure is applied whilst recording video, ECG and EEG. Full cardiopulmonary resuscitation facilities must be available. In susceptible individuals, temporary asystole, with associated increased amplitude and decreased frequency of the EEG tracing, are recorded. Once the heart restarts, the EEG returns to normal.

AUTONOMIC FAILURE (ORTHOSTATIC SYNCOPE)

Whereas in reflex vasovagal syncope there is active vasodilatation and brady-cardia in the face of diminished cardiac output, here failing autonomic function results in reduced or absent vasoconstriction in response to a postural fall in blood pressure.

Clinical features

Syncope occurs within seconds or minutes of assuming the upright posture. Patients are particularly vulnerable on rising and after meals, e.g. in the hour after breakfast. Orthostatic syncope differs from reflex vasovagal syncope in that the skin may be warm, the pulse rate unchanged, and sweating absent.

Risk factors

Several conditions promote orthostatic syncope:

- elderly-related autonomic dysfunction
- medication, especially antihypertensives, phenothiazines, tricyclic anti-depressants, anti-parkinsonian treatments and diuretics
- autonomic neuropathy, especially from diabetes, alcohol and amyloidosis
- complex autonomic failure associated with parkinsonian syndromes such as multiple system atrophy.

Management

- Withdraw any provoking medications.
- Avoid precipitating situations such as prolonged standing, large meals, alcohol and vigorous exercise.
- A head-up tilt at night may help.
- Fludrocortisone acetate (50–200 µg daily) is the usual first-line medication.

CARDIAC SYNCOPE

This refers to syncope associated with cardiac disease: either arrhythmias or structural disorders. Table 4.3 lists the main characteristics of cardiac syncope.

Tachyarrhythmias

A rapid heart rate prevents proper ventricular filling during diastole, thus resulting in pre-syncope and syncope. There is often a history of palpitation both during attacks and at other times. Tachyarrhythmias are either supraventricular or ventricular. Supraventricular tachycardias are more common and are not usually associated with structural heart disease.

Table 4.3
Characteristics of cardiac syncope

- Cardiac syncope is a potentially serious condition with an overall mortality of 30 per cent in the first year

- Exercise-induced syncope requires the urgent exclusion of a cardiac cause. Some exercise-induced syncope is, however, benign, including the normal faint feeling after exercise and the rare variant of reflex vasovagal syncope presenting as exercise-induced syncope

- Cardiac syncope occurs from any posture, and arrhythmogenic syncope is common while in bed

- Cardiac syncope may be misdiagnosed as epilepsy, with potentially fatal consequences. Patients with recurrent syncope or those with a significant family history of syncope should undergo an ECG. Some cases of sudden unexpected death in epilepsy are likely to have been misdiagnosed incidents of cardiac syncope (*see* Chapter 9)

Ventricular tachycardias are more serious and are usually associated with significant heart disease.

Two important inherited conditions, described below, may predispose to tachyarrhythmia.

Wolff–Parkinson–White syndrome

This syndrome shows the ECG characteristics of a short PR interval and a delta wave on the R wave upstroke. This predisposes to 're-entry tachycardias' caused by an abnormal short circuit (the bundle of Kent). The related Lown–Ganong–Levine syndrome is characterized by a short PR interval but no delta wave.

Long QT syndromes

Long QT syndromes are inherited on channel disorders presenting with tachyarrhythmia. The QT interval on the ECG is measured from the peak of the Q wave to the end of the T wave and is corrected for heart rate. The normal corrected value (QT_C = the QT interval divided by the root of the RR interval) is less than 0.46 seconds in males and 0.47 seconds in females. The QT interval normally shortens with increased heart rate, but in the long QT syndromes, there is further QT interval prolongation on exercise.

The cause is a congenitally wide variation in refractoriness between adjacent cardiac myofibrils, causing 'micro re-entry' phenomena. This can lead to the potentially fatal ventricular tachyarrhythmia known as 'torsades de

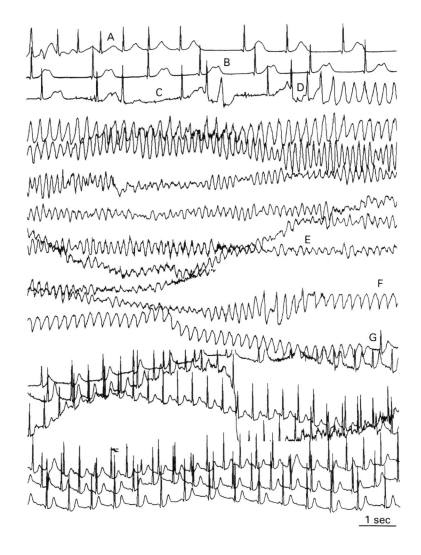

Figure 4.1
Long QT syndrome. ECG showing QT prolongation (A) with giant 'T-wave humps' (B) and short–long RR sequences (C). The arrhythmia begins with an R on T phenomenon (D), followed by torsade de pointes, which deteriorates into ventricular fibrillation (E) and ventricular flutter (F) before reverting to sinus rhythm (G). (Reproduced from Benhorin and Medina, 1997, with permission.)

1 sec

pointes' (Ben-David and Zipes, 1993) (Fig. 4.1), in which the QRS axis repeatedly rotates through 360°.

Genetic long QT syndromes (Viskin, 1999) are associated with abnormalities of either the potassium or the chloride channels. The major phenotypes include the Romano–Ward syndrome (a group of autosomal dominant disorders) and the more severe Jervell and Lange–Neilsen syndrome (autosomal recessive), associated with deafness.

Patients present with recurrent pre-syncope and syncope, particularly after rising in the morning, sometimes progressing to ventricular fibrillation and sudden death. The typical sequence is of falling and lying still for a few seconds before (anoxic) convulsions begin (Singh *et al.*, 1993). This is distinguished from epileptic seizures in which the jerking precedes or coincides with the fall. Anyone, particularly infants or children, presenting with a loss of consciousness following exertion, or recurrent seizures on rising should arouse suspicion of a long QT syndrome.

Acquired QT disorders can be caused by several factors, particularly drugs. Shortening occurs with digoxin, hyperthermia and hypercalcaemia; lengthening occurs with some anti-arrhythmic agents or anti-histamines. Any cardiac disease, particularly ischaemic, may lengthen the QT interval, thus predisposing to arrhythmias.

Bradyarrhythmias

A slow heart rate may result in a cardiac output insufficient to maintain an adequate cerebral circulation, so patients present with fatigue as well as syncope. The most common chronic causes are a complete heart block and sick sinus syndrome. Swallow syncope, in which a bradyarrhythmia occurs as a reflex response to swallowing, is rare and often associated with glosso-pharyngeal neuralgia.

Structural cardiac causes

These lead to syncope by physically impairing cardiac output via three main mechanisms:

- **Left ventricular outflow tract obstruction** is associated with aortic stenosis and hypertrophic obstructive cardiomyopathy. The mechanism of syncope is through reduced stroke volume as well as an increased vagus tone following vigorous ventricular contractions.
- **Left ventricular underfilling** results from mitral stenosis, atrial myxoma or pulmonary hypertension. Again, vigorous contractions contribute to the syncope.
- **Cardiac pump impairment** may occur in cardiomyopathy or ischaemic heart disease. Arrhythmogenic right ventricular dysplasia is an autosomal dominant condition that may present as sudden death. The diagnosis is difficult without a family history since ECG abnormalities (inverted T waves in leads V2–V4) are found in only 70 per cent of cases. At autopsy, the right ventricular wall shows fibrosis, but the patchy process may even be missed on endocardial biopsy.

RESPIRATORY SYNCOPE

In **cough syncope**, vigorous coughing (especially in elderly males) or the performing of the Valsalva manoeuvre (e.g. in trumpet playing) may elevate the intrathoracic pressure sufficiently above venous pressure to impair venous return and cause reflex bradycardia with resulting syncope.

Breath-holding spells are a common source of misdiagnosis in toddlers. Typically, anger, frustration, fear or pain may precipitate two or three loud cries. The breath is held in expiration, and a generalized tonic spasm associated with apnoea follows. Cyanosis is often striking, even before complete apnoea. After a few seconds, breathing restarts and crying resumes. The child may be dazed for about half a minute and then carries on with the interrupted activities. Breath holding is unusual after the age of 3 years. Breath holding (sometimes leading to syncope) may be a feature of Rett syndrome (*see* below).

Hyperventilation must also be considered (*see* below and Chapter 7).

CENTRAL NERVOUS SYSTEM SYNCOPE

Raised intracranial pressure
Raised intracranial pressure may occur intermittently from obstructive hydrocephalus, for example from a third ventricular colloid cyst or a Chiari malformation. There is usually an accompanying generalized 'pressure' headache that may build up over several seconds. The potential result is sudden death.

Autonomic dysreflexia in paraplegia
This is a complication of spinal cord lesions (above T6) so is usually confined to patients with paraparesis and urinary incontinence. A loss of the normal autonomic control of blood pressure allows intermittent massive hypertension, sometimes sufficiently severe to alter consciousness.

Diencephalic attacks
Following diffuse brain insults, for example head injury or hypoxaemia, patients may exhibit intermittent events characterized by hypertension, sweating, tachycardia and even loss of consciousness. These may be confused with seizures but are probably due to ephaptic transmission between damaged axons in the upper brainstem. Diencephalic attacks usually respond well to low-dose carbamazepine.

Concussive (immediate post-traumatic) convulsions
The seizure-like events that may immediately follow a head injury are discussed in Chapter 3.

Behavioural causes

Psychogenic attacks are very important in the differential diagnosis of epilepsy and are considered in detail in Chapter 7.

Hyperventilation from anxiety and panic disorder may culminate in syncope attributable to hyperventilation-induced cerebral vasoconstriction. This is associated with tingling in the finger-tips and face, which may be lateralized. Other symptoms include involuntary curling of the fingers, hands and feet (carpopedal spasm), light-headedness, breathlessness, palpitation, a tight feeling in the chest and throat, blurred vision and feelings of panic.

Psychogenic non-epileptic attack disorder is described in Chapter 7.

The frequent rages in **episodic dyscontrol syndrome** may occasionally be mistaken for epileptic seizures since confusion and aggression are recognized post-ictal phenomena. Post-ictal confusion (*see* Chapter 7) is occasionally cited as a criminal defence. Episodic dyscontrol is distinguished from epilepsy by the history of provocation of individual attacks, whereas seizures are usually spontaneous.

Cerebrovascular disorders

MIGRAINE

Although a migraine aura without headache (migraine equivalent) does occur, a definite diagnosis of migraine requires a clear association with a vascular-type headache and systemic upset, with freedom from symptoms between attacks. Migraine equivalents are generally a diagnosis of exclusion.

The main features that distinguish migraine from seizures are as follows:

- **Visual symptoms.** Typical migraine visual symptoms are zigzag, bright monochrome lights, gradually evolving and moving across the visual field. This is in contrast to visual epilepsy, in which the hallucinations are unformed or circles (but not zigzags), multicoloured and often confined to one half of the visual field (Plate 1) (Panayiotopoulos, 1994).
- **Sensory symptoms.** In migraine, unilateral tingling spreads from one body part to another over 15–30 minutes; it has usually cleared from the first part by the time it reaches the next. This contrasts with a sensory seizure in which symptoms typically spread quickly from one part to involve the entire ipsilateral side, sometimes with convulsion.

Certain migraine variants may be confused with or overlap with epilepsy (Table 4.4).

TRANSIENT ISCHAEMIC ATTACKS

Arteriosclerotic transient ischaemic attacks (TIAs) are broadly distinguished from seizures and migraine by their 'negative' symptoms and retained consciousness.

Table 4.4
Migraine variants caus-
ing diagnostic confusion
with epilepsy

- **Retinal migraine.** This manifests as episodes of unilateral transient visual disturbance, sometimes very frequent, occasionally without headache or systemic upset. Aspirin is an effective prophylaxis

- **Basilar artery migraine.** This is a rare condition occurring in younger patients, presenting as a visual disturbance such as prolonged visual blacking, and brainstem symptoms such as vertigo, double vision and loss of consciousness. Headache and vomiting are usual

- **Migraine syncope.** Gradual loss of consciousness is a rare complication of migraine, particularly familial hemiplegic migraine

- **Migraine–epilepsy syndrome.** There are close links between epilepsy and migraine. A migraine-type headache is a common consequence of an epileptic seizure. Occasional patients with epilepsy describe a migraine-type aura preceding their seizures. The overlap is particularly noticeable in the syndrome of late-onset benign occipital epilepsy (*see* Chapter 3)

- **Migraine coma.** Rarely, coma is attributed to migraine. Often provoked by minor head injury, it proceeds through gradual-onset migraine symptoms to confusion and altered consciousness. The coma may recur, but individual attacks have an excellent prognosis

Negative symptoms such as numbness, weakness or transient blindness contrast with positive symptoms such as tingling and unformed visual hallucination (migraine or seizure) or jerking (seizure). There are notable exceptions to this general rule. Focal jerking accompanies TIAs if bilateral carotid stenosis has severely compromised the cerebral blood flow. Tingling is fairly common in arteriosclerotic TIA. Bilateral visual loss, sometimes lasting many minutes, is characteristic of occipital lobe epilepsy.

Retained consciousness is usual in arteriosclerotic TIAs unless the ischaemia involves the brainstem or the entire cortex (e.g. following hypotension or asystole).

TRANSIENT GLOBAL AMNESIA

This is an unusual condition in which there is transient (several hours) anterograde memory loss characterized by acute amnesia and repeated questioning. This may be accompanied by a migraine-type headache. It has an excellent prognosis and only rarely recurs. It presumably relates to transient ischaemia (vasospasm) of the mesial temporal structures. Recurrent or unusually brief episodes might raise a suspicion of temporal lobe epilepsy, and particularly the form known as transient epileptic amnesia.

Movement disorders

Dystonic, myoclonic and startle disorders are occasionally confused with epilepsy.

DYSTONIA

Paroxysmal dystonias are rare but may mimic seizures:

- **Paroxysmal kinesigenic dystonia.** This is a rare familial condition in which sudden movement provokes involuntary unilateral dystonic posturing lasting a minute or so. It usually responds rapidly to low-dose carbamazepine.
- **Tonic spasms of multiple sclerosis.** These involuntary and sometimes painful unilateral dystonic movements, like other paroxysmal symptoms in multiple sclerosis, respond excellently to carbamazepine.
- **Benign infantile dystonia.** Dystonic episodes may last for hours in otherwise normal infants. Benign paroxysmal torticollis of infancy manifests as episodes of torticollis, with no alteration in consciousness, lasting several hours. The infants are normal between attacks.

MYOCLONIC DISORDERS

- **Hypnic myoclonus** is the normal phenomenon of jerking at sleep onset; its frequency is increased by anxiety and depression.
- **Progressive myoclonic ataxia** is a rare group of disorders in which myoclonus is associated with progressive neurological deficit manifesting as cognitive decline, ataxia and epilepsy.
- **Progressive myoclonic encephalopathy** is caused by a variety of genetic and degenerative conditions and may manifest as non-epileptic myoclonus with impaired cognitive function.
- **Non-epileptic myoclonus in infancy.** In early infancy, benign, non-epileptic myoclonus may occur both during sleep and when awake. Twitching movements may be rhythmic and are unassociated with EEG changes. They may begin when the infant is aged a few days and resolve within a few months. Overall development is normal. In benign

myoclonus of early infancy, runs of spasms occur without EEG accompaniments. The main differential diagnosis is from infantile spasms.

Myoclonus types

Cortical myoclonus

Cortical myoclonus is multifocal and predominantly affects the distal musculature. It is stimulus sensitive (e.g. to tapping the fingers or feet) but not sound sensitive. The EEG may show spike-and-wave activity. The main epileptic causes are myoclonus epilepsy with ragged-red fibres, neuronal ceroid lipofuscinosis, Lafora body disease and Unverricht–Lundbörg disease; the main non-epileptic cause is post-anoxic cortical damage. Treatment is with valproate, clonazepam or piracetam.

Subcortical myoclonus

Subcortical myoclonus is generalized and predominantly affects the proximal musculature. It is stimulus sensitive (e.g. to tapping the face) and markedly sound sensitive. It may be caused by basal ganglia disorders (e.g. benign essential myoclonus), by structural brainstem lesions (e.g. vascular or tumour) or by hereditary hyperekplexia. Treatment is with clonazepam.

Spinal myoclonus

Spinal myoclonus is a rare phenomenon manifesting as involuntary jerking of, for example, a limb or the abdominal musculature. The cause in unknown (investigations are needed to exclude a spinal cord lesion but are usually normal), and the response to medication (e.g. clonazepam) is poor.

STARTLE DISORDERS

An **excessive startle** to a sudden unexpected stimulus may be a variant of normal.

Hyperekplexia (startle disease or 'Jumping Frenchman of Maine') is a rare group of usually familial conditions in which genetic disorders of the glycine receptor lead to susceptibility to startle. Presentation in the neonatal period is with extreme stiffness. The stiffness may fluctuate, suggesting myoclonic or tonic seizures. Misdiagnosis is common but can be fatal since the extreme stiffness may impede breathing and lead to apnoea and death.

OTHER MOVEMENT DISORDERS

Stereotypic behaviour, as seen in mental retardation, may cause diagnostic difficulties, especially in a child who also has seizures.

Rett syndrome, a genetic disorder seen only in girls (being X-linked dominant and lethal in males), manifests with a progressive loss of previously acquired motor and cognitive skills from the age of about 18 months, epilepsy occurring in about 75 per cent of cases. Ambulation is lost, and the purposeful use of the hands becomes replaced by stereotyped activity. Hyperventilation and breath holding are common and may be sufficiently severe to lead to syncope, easily mistaken for seizures.

Sleep disorders

Epileptic seizures may sometimes occur in, or be confined to, sleep so may be confused with non-epileptic sleep-related phenomena.

Narcolepsy

This well-known (and probably overdiagnosed) syndrome presents with excessive daytime somnolence such that sleep may occur in inappropriate situations such as during conversation or meals. Other features include a rapid sleep onset on settling to sleep, poor quality and restless night-time sleep, hypnagogic (just before falling asleep) hallucinations and sleep paralysis. The somnolence is treated with amphetamines or modafinil.

Cataplexy

Cataplexy is part of the narcolepsy syndrome and is the equivalent of rapid eye movement (REM) sleep intruding into wakefulness. It is transient, laughter-induced or emotion-induced axial and facial atonia with dysarthria or mutism, often with facial jerking. There is no altered consciousness. Cataplexy is treated with clomipramine.

Sleep apnoea

This is a common, treatable and under-recognized condition. The associated daytime somnolence may lead to an erroneous diagnosis of epilepsy. Furthermore, the sleep deprivation of sleep apnoea may exacerbate pre-existing epilepsy. Broadly speaking, there are two types:

- In **obstructive sleep apnoea**, sleep-related upper airway collapse leads to frequent apnoeas with sleep fragmentation, poor sleep quality and consequent excessive daytime somnolence. The important predisposing factors are obesity, alcohol and other sedatives, structural upper airway narrowing (including nasal deformity and upper airway congestion) and ventilatory muscle weakness (airway resistance increasing during sleep, leaving the weakened diaphragm unable to cope).
- **Central sleep apnoea.** A disordered control of breathing during sleep may accompany brainstem disorders, resulting in apnoea during sleep ('Ondine's curse').

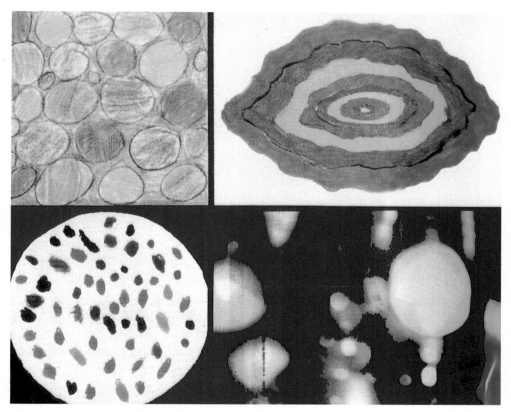

Plate 1 Visual illusions of occipital epilepsy as perceived and illustrated by patients. (Reproduced with permission from Panayiotopoulos, 1994.)

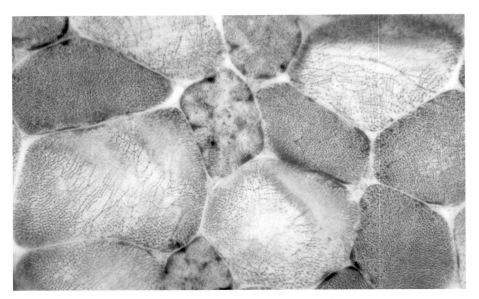

Plate 2 Muscle biopsy (NADH histochemistry) showing subsarcolemmal mitochondrial aggregates ('ragged-red fibres') characteristic of mitochondrial cytopathy.

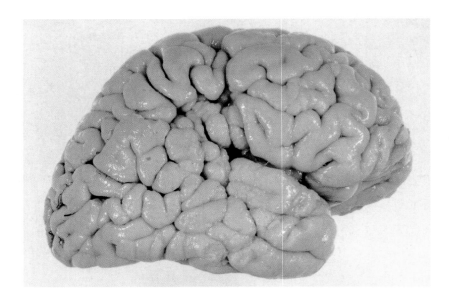

Plate 3 Post-mortem brain: polymicrogyria in the perisylvian region.

Periodic leg movements of sleep

This familial condition is associated with the syndrome of restless legs and manifests as repeated sleep-related myoclonic twitches followed by ankle and hallux extension.

Rapid eye movement sleep behaviour disorder

This results from the dissociation between REM sleep and axial atonia; the patient therefore acts out dreams. It is rare but is particularly seen in the elderly and may result in self-injury. There is often underlying brainstem disease such as multiple sclerosis or multiple system degeneration. Clonazepam is effective.

Night terrors

Night terrors may be confused with nocturnal seizures from frontal lobe epilepsy. The latter have stereotyped motor components, usually with lateralization, and are preceded by a loud cry. Night terrors are likely to cause the child to sit up and scream, apparently unaware of the parents; involuntary motor components are unusual.

Paroxysmal nocturnal dystonia

This condition is now considered synonymous with nocturnal frontal lobe epilepsy rather than being a primary movement disorder, and so the term has been largely abandoned.

Periodic ataxias

These rare autosomal dominant conditions manifest as childhood-onset or adolescent-onset attacks of ataxia, dysarthria, vertigo and nystagmus:

- **Type 1. Episodic ataxia/myokymia**, a potassium channelopathy mapping to chromosome 12p, is the more likely to be confused with epilepsy. It presents with attacks of ataxia and myokymia (muscle rippling) lasting seconds to minutes; the EEG often shows sharp and slow waves. Definite epileptic seizures occur in some cases.
- **Type 2. Acetazolamide-responsive autosomal dominant periodic ataxia**, a calcium channelopathy mapping to chromosome 19p, is closely related to familial hemiplegic migraine and may present as vertigo, ataxia and even blackouts. Acetazolamide is usually an effective treatment.

Vertigo

With a good history, recurrent episodic vertigo should rarely be confused with epilepsy.

Benign paroxysmal positioning vertigo is the most common cause of vertigo in adults: positioning in certain postures provokes transient vertigo and nystagmus.

Ménière's disease also presents as episodic vertigo (attacks lasting 24 minutes to 24 hours) but the progressive unilateral hearing loss provides the diagnosis.

Vertebrobasilar insufficiency is a rare, serious and overdiagnosed cause of vertigo, especially in the elderly. It may herald a posterior circulation infarction. Aspirin is the usual treatment, but if this condition is suspected, it is worth checking the blood pressure in each arm in case of subclavian steal syndrome.

Benign paroxysmal vertigo of childhood occurs around the age of 3–6 years and resolves spontaneously without long-term sequelae. There is a sudden cessation of activity and a look of fear. The child is unsteady and may fall but does not lose consciousness. Nystagmus can be seen, but the child is usually so frightened that his or her face is buried against the carer. Vomiting may occur. Episodes usually last several but less than 30 minutes.

Toxic, metabolic or infectious causes

Hypoglycaemia must be considered in all patients with undiagnosed altered consciousness. The clinical features are listed in Table 4.5. Once thought of, it is easily confirmed and readily reversed.

Table 4.5
The clinical features of hypoglycaemia (from insulinoma)

- Adrenergic features such as hunger, tremulousness, anxiety, sweating, tachycardia and palpitation

- Hypoglycaemic features such as headache, confusion, weakness, behavioural disturbance, seizures and coma

- Loss of consciousness (often with convulsion) occurs especially in the early hours of sleep, i.e. several hours following a meal

- Repeated relief of symptoms by a sweet drink, with subsequent weight gain

- A 72-hour fast may be needed to induce attacks, during which a low blood glucose level and an inappropriately high endogenous insulin level are found

- **Insulin-treated diabetes mellitus** is the most common cause.
- **Insulinoma** may present as recurrent confusion owing to recurrent hypoglycaemia and frequently escapes diagnosis.
- **Organic acid metabolism disorders** may need exclusion in childhood.
- **Other causes.** Hypoglycaemia induced by alcohol, hepatoma or even exogenous insulin (as a feature of Munchausen syndrome) must also be considered.

Although **alcohol** may provoke seizures through toxicity or withdrawal, syncope or coma following alcohol excess may occur as a direct toxic effect and may be exacerbated by hypoglycaemia (*see* Chapter 9)

Illicit drugs are discussed in Chapter 9. It is important to enquire about illicit drug use in patients with an undiagnosed loss of consciousness. Sometimes, however, loss of consciousness may occur in non-drug users who have been deliberately poisoned. Of particular concern are flunitrazepam (Rohypnol) and midazolam, used as 'date-rape drugs'. They dissolve rapidly, are colourless and tasteless, and can induce a trance-like state and muscle relaxation. The associated short-term memory loss makes it harder for rape victims to press charges.

Although unprovoked seizures are uncommon in **porphyria**, acute attacks of confusion and psychosis may mimic epilepsy; inadvertent treatment with anti-epileptic medications such as carbamazepine or phenytoin only exacerbates the porphyria. Porphyria is autosomal dominant so there is usually a family history of psychotic attacks or neuropathy.

Other metabolic disturbances such as hyperammonaemia, ketosis and a high lactate level can produce coma in childhood.

Miscellaneous causes

- **Phaeochromocytoma and carcinoid syndrome.** These may present as attacks of apparent confusion and lead to a misdiagnosis of epilepsy.
- **Suffocation.** In Meadow syndrome (Munchausen syndrome by proxy), the parent, usually the mother, induces illness; suffocation of the child can lead to episodes of anoxia with subsequent jerking similar to that seen in clonic seizures. Covert surveillance may be necessary to confirm the diagnosis.

Age-specific differential diagnosis

The differential diagnoses of epilepsy presenting in different age groups (neonate, infant, young child, teenager and the elderly) are considered in Chapter 9.

Conclusion

The differential diagnosis of seizures and epilepsy is very broad and involves all branches of medicine. A confident diagnosis of epilepsy is essential before anti-epileptic treatment is begun. Where doubt remains, it is usually better to wait for the diagnosis to declare itself more fully.

When and how to investigate

Epileptology is a truly general medical discipline. Not only are there many types of epilepsy, but also there are many conditions that may mimic epilepsy. The importance of correct diagnosis for the appropriate management of people with blackouts cannot be overemphasized.

Clinical aspects

Despite remarkable advances in the technology of imaging and neurophysiology, it is still the clinical features that give the diagnosis. Imaging and neurophysiology tests can supplement, but never substitute for, a detailed history. However, even with an exhaustive history, diagnostic doubt often remains. The clinician must not be rushed into a label of epilepsy; it is better to err towards underdiagnosis than overdiagnosis. An open mind and the passage of time often allow the true nature of the attack to declare itself with fewer problems than accompany a hurried label of epilepsy. Trials of anti-epilepsy treatment are rarely justified in the management of blackouts.

HISTORY TAKING

The key to the diagnosis is the history. The solution to puzzling cases (unusual signs or odd scan appearances) is more often reached by retaking the history than by re-examining the signs or scan.

Presenting complaint

The physician rarely has the privilege of seeing the attacks at first hand but must obtain this information by taking a history from the patient and preferably from an observer. A witness account of the blackout is particularly important and this might involve telephoning a relative or friend from the clinic. The history should include details of the date of first seizure, the seizure types and their frequency, any warning symptoms (aura), the observations of any witness to the attacks, including ictal behaviour, impairment of consciousness, duration of the seizure and post-ictal phenomena. A knowledge of provoking factors and changes with maturation is also important.

Other epilepsy history

Having described the main symptoms, it is usual to ask directly for a history of previous tonic-clonic seizures, episodes of status, absence attacks, myoclonus and photosensitivity.

Medication

Patients with long-standing epilepsy have often tried several anti-epileptic medications, so the history should include details of present and past anti-epileptic medication, documenting the drug name (including the brand name), the maximum dose, the effects and side effects and, if appropriate, the reasons for discontinuation.

Often, a patient has tried a drug that has failed to control the seizures, but tried it at a suboptimal dose, leaving the potential to try the same drug again. Combinations of drugs (polypharmacy) should be noted since a drug's failure can sometimes be attributed to its interactions. Some idea of compliance with medication should be obtained. Other medications should also be recorded as these may themselves provoke seizures or interact with anti-epileptic medication.

Past and birth history

In patients of all ages with epilepsy, it is useful to obtain a birth and early life history since causative factors are often identified. Problems with the pregnancy, birth or early development, or the occurrence of febrile convulsions, may be relevant to the subsequent epilepsy history. A history of significant head injury (with loss of consciousness or skull fracture), meningitis or encephalitis, drug or toxin exposure and other central nervous system or systemic illnesses should be specifically sought. Details of psychiatric illness should also be asked for.

Family history

Details of other family members with epilepsy should be obtained. This information is often surprisingly incomplete as an epilepsy history is commonly concealed from relatives. It can be useful to retake the family history once a definite diagnosis of an epileptic attack has been made for the patient. Many types of epilepsy are now known to have a genetic association, making the family history an important aspect of history taking.

Social history

The patient's occupation, employment status, education history and domestic situation (including the receipt of state invalidity benefits) are important. Is the patient driving? If the seizures are poorly controlled, are there other safety issues? Alcohol intake should also be documented.

A suggested outline for history taking in a patient presenting with seizures is presented in Table 5.1

Seizure localization

From the history, or if a seizure is witnessed or recorded on video, some inferences about the seizure localization can be drawn (Table 5.2).

PHYSICAL EXAMINATION

All new patients presenting with blackouts must undergo a physical examination, with particular emphasis on the cardiovascular, neurological and dermatological systems:

- **General examination** should include a search for signs of neurocutaneous syndromes (neurofibromas, scalp haemangioma or the stigmata of tuberous sclerosis), dysmorphic features and scalp scars.
- **Cardiovascular examination** is especially important if the history suggests a syncopal origin. The heart rate, heart rhythm and heart sounds, as well as measuring of the lying and standing blood pressure and pulse rate, are important. The blood pressure measurement in each arm may differ, suggesting subclavian steal syndrome, one of the few treatable causes of vertebrobasilar ischaemia.
- **Neurological examination** should include assessing the patient's visual fields and optic disc appearance, listening over the orbits for a cerebral bruit and searching for lateralizing signs. Subtle signs such as pathological left-handedness, evidence of body size asymmetry (hemismallness in the limbs or mild facial asymmetry), mirror movements or an impairment of fine motor skills can all be important.

It is actually quite unusual to find significant neurological signs in patients presenting with epilepsy; extra history taking while examining is often more rewarding.

> The diagnosis of epilepsy rests mainly on the history and less on test results.

Table 5.1
History details for patients with seizures or probable seizures

General information

| Seen alone or with a witness | Age |
| Right or left handed |

Seizure description (for each seizure type)

Age at seizure onset	
Time of day	Post-ictal symptoms
Situation	Tongue biting
Warning	Incontinence
Consciousness retained?	Injury
Colour	Frequency
Jerking	Date of last event
Lateralized symptoms	Provoking factors
Duration	

Specifically enquire about

| Myoclonic jerks | Photosensitivity |
| Absences | Episodes of status epilepticus |

Anti-epileptic medication

| Present medication (including brand name and dosing frequency) | Previous medication (including dose and reason for stopping) |

Past medical history

Other significant illness	Head injury (duration of retrograde amnesia, loss of
Birth	consciousness, skull fracture,
Febrile convulsions	duration of post-traumatic
Cerebral infection (meningitis, encephalitis)	amnesia, intracranial haematoma, neurosurgery)
	Depression, anxiety symptoms, psychosis
	Learning disability

Family history

| Of epilepsy | Of other significant disorders |

Social history

Schooling	Alcohol
Work	Illicit drugs
Living with whom?	Driving
Hobbies and interests	

- **Epigastric aura** strongly suggests a medial temporal lobe focus

- **Déjà vu** usually suggests a dominant hemisphere temporal focus

- **Head turning** (aversion) prior to a tonic-clonic seizure localizes to the opposite frontal lobe

- **Dystonic posturing** of a limb (e.g. the elevation of one arm, finger spreading) almost always localizes to the opposite hemisphere

- **Automatisms** are usually bilateral (e.g. lip smacking, hand wringing); if unilateral (e.g. rubbing), they are commonly ipsilateral to the epileptic focus

- **Aphasia** at seizure onset suggests a dominant hemisphere focus

- **Ictal speech** suggests a focus in the non-dominant hemisphere

- **Ictal vomiting** is associated with right temporal lobe localization

- **Ictal fear** localizes to the amygdala

- **Post-ictal hemiparesis** (Todd's paresis) or hemianaesthesia localizes to the opposite hemisphere

- **Post-ictal aphasia** suggests a dominant hemisphere lesion

Table 5.2
Localizing value of manifestations of epileptic seizures

Investigation of epilepsy

Unlike conditions such as diabetes or anaemia, there is, for the most part, no 'diagnostic test' for epilepsy. Investigations such as an EEG or brain scan may refine the clinical conclusion, but the diagnosis remains essentially clinical.

THE EEG

What is an EEG?

Electroencephalography involves the detection, amplification, filtering, display, storage and analysis of small changes in electrical potential produced by the brain, mostly the underlying cortex (Fish, 1995). Recordings are made with electrodes in specific scalp locations and with leads displayed in a variety of predetermined patterns (montages).

Routine (interictal) recording

A routine EEG recording takes 20–30 minutes during which the patient is initially resting but awake and is then activated by overbreathing for 2–3 minutes and exposed to flashing lights at various frequencies (photic stimulation). It is helpful to videotape the procedure in case specific events occur during the recording. Special techniques might include making recordings during sleep, during normal activities (ambulatory recordings) or with videotape over a prolonged period, including sleep.

Limitations of the EEG

The EEG is much over-rated as a diagnostic tool for blackouts by both patients and some doctors. Those who have been impressed by its apparent complexity and mystique often receive the knowledge of its limitations with surprise and disappointment. The EEG is open to over-reporting and the misinterpretation of minor changes. Undue emphasis placed upon 'suspicious' EEGs is repeatedly the cause of misdiagnosis of epilepsy.

The normal EEG is strikingly age dependent and varies considerably between individuals. During infancy and childhood, rhythms are slower, and some excess of slow activity may persist into adolescence.

In addition, the EEG may be normal in epilepsy. Only 30 per cent of adults undergoing a routine EEG at an interval following a definite seizure (which varies with the age group and clinical characteristics) show abnormalities definitely in keeping with an epilepsy tendency, i.e. spike-and-wave activity. A further 30 per cent have abnormalities that are suggestive but non-specific, for example lateralized sharpened slow waveforms, and 30 per cent are normal. Thus, a report stating 'compatible with epilepsy' is actually applicable to any EEG record (Mathews, 1975).

> The EEG is often normal in people with epilepsy. It is not a 'test' for epilepsy.

An important factor influencing the EEG report is the clinical information provided to the neurophysiologist. Unless this information is comprehensive, the EEG report will be devalued. Information such as 'blackout query cause' is unlikely to generate a particularly helpful EEG report.

Indications

To support an epilepsy diagnosis

In a patient suspected of having epilepsy, an EEG is a useful adjunct to the clinical diagnosis. Finding definite spike-and-wave epileptiform activity is clearly very helpful. Sharp waves are less conclusive, but an abnormal excess of such findings, particularly if focal, will be helpful. An EEG immediately after a seizure usually shows a post-ictal slowing of brain rhythms, either focal or generalized; this is a useful test in distinguishing seizures from non-epileptic attacks.

Despite its clear benefits, the EEG still has significant limitations in diagnosing epilepsy; considerable caution is needed in EEG interpretation for several reasons.

The EEG may be normal in people with unequivocal epilepsy

This is not surprising since an EEG is limited by both temporal factors (20–30 minutes recording when the seizures may be occurring monthly) and spatial factors (surface recording missing deep foci). Only if a typical event is captured upon EEG – a relatively uncommon occurrence during a 20-minute standard interictal recording – does the EEG secure the diagnosis of epilepsy. Even then, simple partial seizures, especially from deep midline frontal foci, may not be associated with abnormal surface EEG activity.

The EEG may show spike-and-wave in people who do not have epilepsy

Finding spike-and-wave 'epileptic' activity does not necessarily mean that the patient's attacks are epileptic. For example, in patients with a known underlying structural lesion, such as cerebral palsy, localized 'epileptiform' EEG changes can occur that are not necessarily associated with seizure activity. Also, following craniotomy, the skull 'window' allows rhythms that appear abnormal, for example sharp waves, but that have no epileptiform significance, to be recorded by scalp electrodes.

To assess the epilepsy type

An important role of the EEG is to distinguish generalized from localization-related epilepsy since the treatment of each is different. Figure 5.1 shows the interictal EEG of a patient with a focal brain lesion. When abnormalities are found, the distinction between generalized or focal spike-and-wave activity is usually easy. Again, however, there might be problems:

- Some partial onset seizures rapidly generalize, giving the EEG appearance of a generalized onset. This is particularly likely in medial frontal seizures owing to the intimate connections of one frontal lobe with the other.
- Some generalized seizures show asymmetry of surface EEG activity.
- Some patients have both generalized and partial seizures.

To identify photosensitivity

Finding photosensitivity is important as it may influence both diagnosis and management. It is especially likely in children and adolescents, amongst

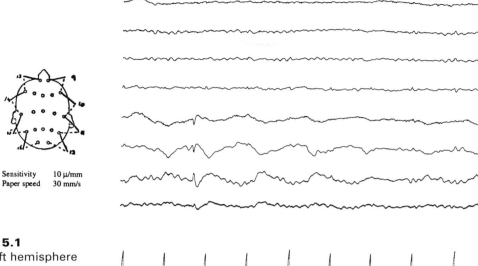

Figure 5.1
EEG: left hemisphere focus (slow waves and spikes).

Sensitivity   10 µ/mm
Paper speed   30 mm/s

whom 10 per cent of patients presenting with a first seizure, particularly females, have unequivocal photosensitivity.

EEG testing is performed at several flash frequencies, each with the eyes open and then closed (as the response may vary with each). The finding of generalized spike-and-wave during exposure to flashing lights is unequivocal and strongly associated with a history of epilepsy; lesser findings, for example occipital or parieto-occipital spikes, are merely suggestive.

To support a syndrome diagnosis

A diagnosis of typical absences requires typical EEG findings of three per second spike-and-wave activity (*see* Fig. 2.1). For other epilepsy syndromes, the information on the EEG is less specific but may support the clinical suspicion. Benign childhood epilepsy with centrotemporal spikes, for example, has a characteristic EEG pattern (*see* Fig. 3.2) only rarely mimicked by underlying structural lesions.

To help in epilepsy prognosis

The EEG is not very good at making a prediction of epilepsy outcome. A patient with epilepsy and an abnormal EEG may never again experience a seizure, whereas some patients with repeatedly normal EEGs go on to have frequent attacks. Nevertheless, following a single seizure (at least in children), spike-and-wave activity on the EEG is helpful in predicting seizure recurrence (Stroink *et al.*, 1998). In addition, an abnormal EEG is an adverse prognostic factor for seizure recurrence following anti-epileptic drug withdrawal (MRC, 1991a).

Ictal recording

If the history does not give the diagnosis and the standard EEG fails to provide diagnostic information, an attempt to record the EEG during seizures may be considered.

Routine EEG with video

It is a great advantage to see attacks as well as to examine the EEG tracing during them. A useful technique is to record on to video every EEG. Seizures captured during the recording can then be observed and analysed in detail afterwards. Recordings on which no seizures are captured can later be erased. More prolonged recordings, for example 4–8 hours, have a greater chance of capturing attacks; a video ensures that these can be assessed in detail at a later time.

Ambulatory EEG

Method   Recording electrodes are attached to the scalp, the wiring being scarcely visible under normal hair. A portable recorder is worn on a belt. The patient completes a diary of activity, a button event marker allowing the recording to be correlated to specific events.

Indication   The technique is particularly useful for young children and for people with learning disability in whom there is difficulty in assessing the frequency and nature of attacks from the history. In addition, once the monitor is in position, it may be possible to gain greater cooperation with recording than during a routine EEG. In adult practice, however, ambulatory monitoring frequently proves disappointing in determining the nature of undiagnosed blackouts.

Advantages   Ambulatory EEG has the advantage of recording seizures in the patient's natural environment and is especially useful if a patient is having frequent undiagnosed attacks, for example more than two per week. A simultaneous ECG recording is useful, not only to see arrhythmias resulting from seizures, but also to detect a cardiac cause of the blackouts, such as complete heart block or supraventricular tachycardia.

Drawbacks   There are several disadvantages to the technique:

- The clinician cannot see what the patient looked like during any events captured on the recording.

- The number of leads available for recording is limited by practical constraints.
- Movement artefacts during events may leave diagnostic doubt.

It is particularly unwise to make a positive diagnosis of non-epileptic attacks from such a recording without an accompanying video recording.

Video EEG

Method   The patient wears a full montage of EEG leads, is confined to a video-recording room and is asked to remain within camera range. A split screen enabling a simultaneous view of the video and the EEG recordings is very helpful, allowing a close correlation between clinical and EEG events.

Advantages   Seizure observation on video is extremely helpful in the diagnosis of epilepsy. The gold standard method of seizure recording is with video and simultaneous EEG recording. As this facility becomes more widely available, it is replacing ambulatory recording as the preferred method of prolonged EEG recording.

Drawbacks   Its main disadvantages are that such inpatient resources are limited and often available only in specialist centres, and that the patients are confined in an unnatural environment.

EEG brain mapping

Method   Brain mapping involves the generation of brain images from the EEG tracing, making the EEG more meaningful to the non-specialist.

Advantages   The particular advantage is in highlighting subtle abnormalities, which might otherwise have passed unnoticed on the ordinary EEG tracing.

Disadvantages   No new information is provided, and brain maps must be interpreted with caution. Pictures generated without proper heed to the correct setting of controls, montages and references, or without a proper appreciation of the influence of biological factors (such as sleep deprivation and immaturity) on the EEG can lead to gross misinterpretation (Binnie and MacGillivray, 1992). It is possible to generate visually pleasing and seemingly credible pictures in which the 'abnormality' is entirely artefactual. An essential precaution is that a standard EEG accompanies every brain map and that the EEG is seen as the standard. A brain map is blind without the EEG (Duffy, 1986).

Invasive EEG monitoring

Indication   These procedures are limited to patients with localization-related epilepsy who are being considered for epilepsy surgery.

Advantages   The EEG recording quality can be greatly enhanced by placing the recording electrode nearer to or in the brain, thereby overcoming the artefact and attenuation of EEG signals passing through the skull and scalp. Such techniques have highlighted the unreliability of the surface EEG, both interictally and even ictally, in localizing the site of seizure origin.

Method   Electrodes are targeted at the supposed epileptogenic zone. There are four grades of depth electrode recording; in general, the more invasive the technique, the better the quality and extent of recording, but the greater the complication risk.

   Foramen ovale electrodes are inserted percutaneously beneath the medial zygoma through the foramen ovale to lie beneath the dura at the base of the medial temporal lobe. With only a limited recording area, the technique is applicable only when there is a high likelihood of a medial temporal seizure origin.

   Epidural electrode placement involves an intermediate level of invasiveness since the dura is still not penetrated. Electrodes are passed through the skull but still lie outside the dura in positions corresponding to the surface EEG electrodes. This technique is best suited to recording from the brain convexity rather than from the base of the temporal lobe.

   Subdural electrode recording (electrocorticography) involves the insertion of electrodes through a burr hole to penetrate the dura and positioning them on the brain's surface. A whole grid of electrodes can be placed on the cortex by full craniotomy. There is inevitably a higher risk of bleeding and local infection than when the dura is left intact.

   Intracerebral electrode recording (depth EEG recording) involves the stereotactic insertion of electrodes into any part of the brain, although more eloquent areas and major arterial territories are usually avoided. The procedure is best suited to recording from the hippocampus or the nearby amygdala, the most common sources of partial seizures.

BRAIN IMAGING

There are two main reasons to image the brain in patients with epilepsy:

1. **To establish a cause for the seizures**, preferably a treatable one. Pathologies such as mesial temporal sclerosis, hippocampal atrophy, malformations (particularly cortical dysplasias), tumours, vascular and

traumatic lesions might each require specific treatment. Improved brain imaging methods have resulted in an improved understanding of the causes of epilepsy, with a consequently better application of potentially curative epilepsy surgery.

2. **To aid classification of the epilepsy,** thus enabling accurate information, for example on prognosis, to be provided to patients and their families.

The brain may be imaged either structurally or functionally.

Structural imaging

Computed tomography

Computed tomography (CT) brain scanning is readily accessible and convenient but does involve radiation exposure, and so is invasive. It can identify gross lesions responsible for epilepsy, for example brain tumour, stroke and tuberous sclerosis. It is particularly good for looking at calcified lesions or skull abnormalities such as fractures. However, CT scanning frequently misses epileptogenic structural lesions such as hippocampal sclerosis, low-grade tumours, hamartomas, cavernomas and cortical dysplasias. In the detailed investigation of epilepsy, therefore, CT scanning has now been replaced by magnetic resonance imaging (MRI).

Magnetic resonance imaging

MRI is the structural imaging method of choice in epilepsy (ILAE Neuroimaging Commission, 1997). T1-weighted and T2-weighted images of the whole brain using minimal slice thickness should be obtained. The images should be reported by a specialist neuroradiologist or experienced clinician, and interpreted in the light of the entire clinical situation.

Improvements in MRI technology have allowed a probable structural basis for localization-related epilepsy to be identified in some 80 per cent of cases (Li *et al.*, 1995), although only a minority of these are surgically resectable. Examples of potentially surgically treatable epileptogenic lesions visible on MRI but not on CT are as follows (*see* Chapter 3):

- mesial temporal sclerosis
- dysembryoplastic neuroepithelial tumour
- ganglioglioma
- cavernoma
- malformations of cortical development.

MRI or CT?

MR scanning is the preferred method of brain imaging for three main reasons:

1. It is considerably more sensitive to the lesions that may cause epilepsy.
2. It provides a much more detailed picture of the brain anatomy and the extent and localization of the lesion.
3. It does not involve radiation exposure.

Owing to present scarcity of resources, however, CT scanning is still often the more practical first-line brain imaging procedure.

Who should be scanned?

Brain imaging, preferably by MRI, is indicated in the majority of patients with a recent spontaneous single seizure or newly diagnosed epilepsy. Patients with a definite diagnosis of generalized epilepsy do not require imaging unless there are special features. MRI is particularly indicated for those in whom any of the following apply:

- A partial-onset seizure has occurred or is suspected at any age. This includes partial seizures with secondary generalization.
- The onset of epilepsy of any type has occurred either in the first years of life or in adulthood, i.e. aged over 20 years. Generalized epilepsy with an onset in children or teenagers does not usually require imaging. If a completely confident diagnosis of benign epilepsy of childhood with centrotemporal spikes (BECTS) can be made, imaging is not necessary.
- There are focal neurological signs.
- There are focal abnormalities on the EEG.
- The epilepsy proves refractory to first-line anti-epileptic medication.
- A loss of control or a change in seizure pattern occurs.

Functional imaging

Single photon emission computed tomography

Single photon emission computed tomography (SPECT) scanning is widely available and can help in seizure localization in localization-related epilepsy. Following an injection of radiolabelled tracer, an image of the brain's uptake of the tracer can be computed. Regional cerebral perfusion can be mapped using tracers such as hexamethyl-propylene-amine-oxime.

SPECT in epilepsy is broadly divided into interictal and peri-ictal studies. **Interictal SPECT** is easy to perform and can be carried out at any time in relation to seizures. Hypoperfusion of the epileptogenic zone is found in 50–80 per cent of cases (Duncan R, 1997).

Ictal (or peri-ictal) SPECT is much more difficult as the injection must be made at the time of a seizure; it demonstrates hyperperfusion of the epileptogenic zone in 70–90 per cent of cases. Ictal SPECT is particularly useful in providing support to the localization of the epileptogenic zone when planning epilepsy surgery in patients without gross anatomical lesions. It is also useful in defining which part of a large lesion is epileptogenic, bringing the possibility of surgery to patients with otherwise apparently unresectable lesions. Ictal SPECT is difficult in frontal seizures, in which there may be little or no aura and only a brief seizure. Ictal SPECT recordings can sometimes replace depth EEG recordings (avoiding an invasive procedure) in patients with mesial temporal sclerosis.

Positron emission tomography

Positron emission tomography (PET) scanning is expensive and limited to only a few specialist centres. It has frequently proved very useful in planning epilepsy surgery. However, with advances in MRI (especially functional MRI) and because of the radiation dose involved, its place in epilepsy assessment will become more limited in future.

As with SPECT, PET scanning involves injecting radiolabelled material that is taken up by the brain, allowing the imaging of the radioactive particles emitted from the sites of uptake. PET imaging has far more applications than SPECT. As well as being able to map cerebral blood flow (using ^{15}O-labelled water), PET can also map regional glucose metabolism (^{18}F-deoxyglucose) as well as the distribution of certain receptors (e.g. using ^{11}C-flumazenil) (Duncan J, 1997).

Almost all PET studies of epilepsy are interictal, demonstrating an area of hypometabolism in and around the epileptogenic zone. PET scan changes do not identify the underlying aetiology, and detailed MRI is still necessary.

Functional MRI

This rapidly developing and promising technique uses the state of haemoglobin oxygenation to image brain function. An excess of deoxygenated haemoglobin occurring in a brain region with increased oxygen uptake can be imaged. It therefore provides a radiation-free method of functional imaging. It can already reliably localize hand motor function. Cognitive changes as well as memory functions may soon be reliably imaged, giving hope that functional MRI will come to replace the Wada test in the presurgery evaluation of epilepsy.

Magnetoencephalography

This imaging technique is based upon the principle that as a 'current' flows down an axon, a tiny magnetic field is generated around it. The brain's natural magnetic field is infinitesimally small, about a billionth that of the Earth. It can be detected only by using semi-conducting quantum interference devices, which convert the magnetic field to a current and then to an output voltage; using an array of sensors, a magnetic field map can be constructed. When the signals are superimposed upon an MR image (magnetic source imaging), the three-dimensional characteristics of an epileptogenic focus can be characterized (Hummel and Stefan, 1997).

Magnetoencephalography has proved promising in localizing epileptogenic foci more accurately than standard EEG imaging or even PET scanning. This is partly because magnetic fields pass unimpeded and unattenuated through the skull and scalp.

The equipment is expensive and bulky, and requires the maintenance of the superconductors at a very low temperature (e.g. minus 269 °C). Unfortunately, therefore, the technique remains little used in practice.

OTHER INVESTIGATIONS

Home video recording of seizures
It is always best to try to see events rather than just having to rely upon the account of the patient and witness. Lending the parent, partner or carer a video camera makes for a very efficient use of resources in diagnosing blackouts.

Cardiovascular investigations
Because syncope is often mistaken for epileptic seizures (*see* Chapter 4), it is important to consider the need for cardiovascular investigations in patients presenting with epilepsy. This is particularly important if the seizure is provoked by exertion, emotion or an upright posture, or is associated with marked pallor or sweating, or where the jerking movements begin only after a few seconds of unconsciousness (*see* Chapter 4).

Electrocardiogram
A standard resting ECG can sometimes detect a predisposition to important arrhythmias (*see* Chapter 4):

- **bradycardias**, including various degrees of conduction block, for example bifascicular or complete heart block;
- **tachyarrhythmias**, especially supraventricular, for example paroxysmal atrial tachycardia;
- **re-entry syndromes** with a short PR interval such as Wolff–Parkinson–White syndrome and Lown–Ganong–Levine syndrome;
- **long QT syndromes**, for example Romano–Ward syndrome or the Jervell and Lange–Nielson syndrome.

As with the EEG and epilepsy, however, a normal ECG does not exclude a cardiogenic cause for syncope. The diagnosis of long QT syndromes, for example, may require an exercise ECG.

Tilt table

The tilt table test has proved useful in the detection of a tendency towards vasovagal and orthostatic syncope. The patient is upright but tilted back at 60 degrees so that the leg muscles are not weight bearing and the blood may pool passively with gravity. This posture is maintained for about 45 minutes. Susceptible patients will show a fall in blood pressure and paradoxical fall in pulse rate and may lose consciousness in a faint. Tilting shows a high sensitivity (up to 90 per cent) and specificity (70 per cent) for a syncopal tendency. It is therefore particularly useful when syncope is suspected but other clinical evidence is lacking (e.g. there is an unwitnessed blackout in the bathroom at night).

For patients with a negative test, syncope may be induced in susceptible individuals using isoprenaline. This increases the sensitivity and shortens the duration of the test but unfortunately gives a less specific result, so is arguably less useful.

Polygraphic recordings

Monitoring the ventilation and blood oxygenation may sometimes be useful in investigating undiagnosed blackouts. Obstructive sleep apnoea may be sufficiently severe to mimic epileptic seizures. In some seizures, the breathing disturbance (e.g. apnoea) is a prominent and an alarming component of the seizure. Furthermore, sleep apnoea may itself exacerbate a seizure tendency through sleep deprivation.

Polygraphic recordings are cumbersome and difficult, however, and, with regard to epilepsy, remain largely a research tool. Where recordings have been made, surprisingly marked autonomic accompaniments of epileptic seizures are occasionally identified (Nashef *et al.*, 1996).

Blood tests

In newly presenting patients with blackouts, certain blood tests, for example glucose, calcium and prolactin, preferably taken at the time of the blackout, may help.

The first test in any patient found unexpectedly confused or unconscious must be a blood **glucose**. Hypoglycaemia is a much rarer cause of altered consciousness than epilepsy, but the consequences of prolonged hypoglycaemia are much more serious; it is a diagnosis not to be missed.

Hypocalcaemia (and less commonly hypercalcaemia) should be considered in undiagnosed blackouts.

The level of blood **prolactin** increases following a seizure, particularly a tonic-clonic seizure. This test can therefore be used to provide support for a clinical diagnosis of a seizure; if normal, it may suggest that the apparent seizure was not epileptic. The blood for prolactin should be taken 20 minutes after the seizure onset. False negatives and positives occur, and so an excessive reliance on the test is unjustified.

Metabolic aspects

Some epilepsies, which are strongly associated with metabolic disturbances, are described in Chapter 3.

Inborn errors of metabolism

The seizures usually start in the neonatal or early infantile period, but some intermittent metabolic upsets, such as fatty acid oxidation defects, can precipitate seizures at a later time. The attacks are likely to be either myoclonic or tonic, but other seizure types may occur. Delayed development, poor hair growth, skin disorders, abdominal organomegaly and prolonged post-ictal coma should all raise the possibility of an underlying error of metabolism. Suggested investigations are listed in Table 5.3.

Acquired metabolic disorders

- **General medical.** Hypoglycaemia and hyponatraemia and hypernatraemia often arise secondary to medical treatment.
- **Renal.** Acute or chronic renal failure is accompanied by seizures in approximately one-third of cases. Both uraemia and the encephalopathy that can be associated with dialysis may be responsible.
- **Hepatic.** Seizures complicate hepatic encephalopathy in less than one-third of patients. In cirrhosis, alcohol withdrawal may be a more potent precipitant than liver disease.
- **Hypocalcaemia**, which is sufficient to cause seizures, is most often found following thyroid or parathyroid surgery.
- **Anoxic–ischaemic insults** to the brain commonly precipitate seizures.
- **Alcohol.** Alcohol and other drugs of abuse must be considered in the differential of causes of acute symptomatic seizures. Most alcohol-related seizures occur in the first 72 hours after cessation of the use of alcohol. Alcoholics are, in addition, likely to have seizures in association with cerebrovascular accidents, which may be minor, and following unrecognized head injuries.
- **Other drugs of abuse** (*see* Chapter 9).

Genetic aspects

An inherited basis for epilepsy has been suspected since the time of Hippocrates. Clear evidence for a genetic basis for epilepsy is seen in about 20 per cent of epilepsy patients, especially children with idiopathic epilepsies. In fact, the majority of epilepsies seem to have some genetic contribution. Patients labelled as having cryptogenic epilepsy can often be shown to have

Table 5.3
Metabolic investigation
in epilepsy

Disorder	Metabolic test
Neonatal period	
Pyridoxine dependency	Test dose of intravenous pyridoxine
Hypoglycaemia	Blood glucose
Hypocalcaemia	Blood calcium
Hypomagnesaemia	Blood magnesium
Urea cycle disorder	Blood ammonia
Amino acid disorders including non-ketotic hyperglycinaemia	Blood, urine and CSF amino acids
Organic acidurias	Urine organic acids
Pyruvate dehydrogenase and other deficiencies of enzymes in the Krebs' cycle	Blood (and CSF) lactate
Molybdenum co-factor deficiency	Uric acid, sulphite oxidase
Peroxisomal disorders	Very long-chain fatty acids
Later infancy and childhood	
Amino acid disorders	Amino acids, as above
Organic acidurias	Organic acids, as above
Fatty acid oxidation defects	Organic acids
Lysosomal storage disorders	Specific lysosomal enzymes
Peroxisomal disorders	Very long-chain fatty acids
Mitochondrial disorders	Blood and CSF lactate
Molybdenum co-factor deficiency	Uric acid, sulphite oxidase
Menkes' disease	Copper, caeruloplasmin
Glucose transporter deficiency	Blood and CSF glucose
Biotinidase deficiency	Serum biotinidase
Porphyria	Urinary porphyrins
Intermittent ataxia with epilepsy	Electrolytes (genetic testing)
Carbohydrate-deficient glycoprotein syndrome	Serum disialotransferrin
Sialidosis	Urinary oligosaccharides

MRI evidence of congenital developmental disorders with a strong likelihood of a genetic basis. Even patients with apparently purely acquired epilepsy, such as that following a stroke, appear more likely than the general population to have a family history of epilepsy.

Although it is common to find a family history of epilepsy or febrile seizures in patients presenting with seizure disorders, it is rare to find epilepsy inherited in a simple (Mendelian) fashion such as autosomal dominant, recessive or X-linked inheritance. Positional cloning and positional candidate techniques are now enabling the construction of the beginnings of an epilepsy gene map, but genetic tests are at present applicable only to a very small proportion of epilepsies.

The genetic basis of epilepsy falls into three categories (Berkovic and Scheffer, 1999):

1. epilepsy as one part of a single-gene (Mendelian) disorder
2. epilepsy as the only manifestation of a single-gene (Mendelian) disorder
3. epilepsy with complex (polygenic) inheritance.

Epilepsy as part of a single-gene disorder

There are hundreds of rare conditions with single-gene (Mendelian) inheritance in which epilepsy is just one manifestation. These inherited symptomatic epilepsies are, however, rare, accounting for a tiny minority of epilepsy patients. Genetic linkage and a molecular basis have been established for many of these conditions. Most are associated with significant neurological impairment and learning disability. Particularly important are the neuronal migration disorders (*see* Chapter 3), increasingly recognized to underlie a significant proportion of epilepsy and learning disability. Unfortunately, knowledge of the genetic basis of these single-gene disorders has had little impact on the understanding of the genetics of epilepsy in general.

Single-gene disorders may be inherited in a number of ways:

- **Autosomal dominant.** Examples include neurocutaneous syndromes such as tuberous sclerosis (*see* Chapter 3), familial cavernomas and familial periventricular heterotopias (filamin 1 mutations).
- **X-linked.** These disorders include X-linked lissencephaly with double-cortex syndrome (abnormal 'doublecortin' protein), Rett syndrome and fragile X syndrome.
- **Autosomal recessive.** Examples include the progressive myoclonic epilepsies, for example Unverricht–Lundbörg disease (cystatin B gene mutations), Lafora body disease (tyrosine phosphatase mutations) and late infantile ceroid lipofuscinosis.
- **Mitochondrial.** The best-known mitochondrial cytopathy causing epilepsy is myoclonic epilepsy with ragged-red fibres.

Epilepsy as the only manifestation of a single-gene disorder

A few rare epilepsies show single-gene inheritance, and this is where the first successes in epilepsy gene identification have been achieved. There are many inherited idiopathic epilepsy syndromes, and it seems likely that a very large number of genes will eventually be identified as causing them. Most of the conditions so far identified result from mutations within ion channel genes.

Even within a family in which epilepsy is inherited by a single abnormal gene, there may be considerable clinical heterogeneity. The epilepsy might appear to have skipped generations. Some family members may have only a mild disorder such as a history of febrile convulsions, whereas others may have a severe form of epilepsy with learning disability; the majority have epilepsy of intermediate severity. As with any genetic disorder, the gene(s) responsible for the family's epilepsy may, through an interaction with other (susceptibility) genes and with the environment, express themselves differently within a family.

The epilepsy syndromes in which single-gene inheritance has been confirmed are described below.

Benign familial neonatal convulsions   In this condition, generalized seizures characteristically occur in otherwise normal neonates from the third day of life. Seizures may recur over several weeks but persist into later life only in about 10 per cent of cases. Most cases are linked to chromosome 20q (gene *KCNQ2*), with some mapping to 8q (*KCNQ3*). These are potassium channel genes; their abnormality allows sodium and calcium channels to predominate and thus allow excess neuronal excitation. Interestingly, *KCNQ1*, a similar gene but expressed in the heart and ear, is mutated in some families with the long QT syndrome.

Benign familial infantile convulsions   This is a localization-related epilepsy in which seizures begin between the ages of 4 and 7 months, and usually settle spontaneously. It is genetically distinct from benign familial neonatal convulsions. Some families show a linkage to chromosome 19q or chromosome 6. In the latter case, there is a tendency for patients to develop paroxysmal choreoathetosis typically around age 10 years, strongly suggesting an ion channel aetiology.

Autosomal dominant nocturnal frontal lobe epilepsy   This is a relatively common and important epilepsy syndrome (*see* Chapter 3) and was the first epilepsy affecting adults to be characterized genetically. The usual age of seizure onset is in childhood, at around the age of 10 years, but it persists into adulthood (Scheffer *et al.*, 1995). The seizures are usually confined to sleep.

The first described kindred showed a single missense mutation in the gene *CHRNA4* coding for the α-4 subunit of the neuronal nicotinic acetylcholine receptor on chromosome 20q. These receptors regulate the release of certain neurotransmitters, including glutamate and dopamine. However, this mutation is actually quite rare. Most families show a linkage to chromosome

15q (Oldani *et al.*, 1998). Both mutations may impair intracellular calcium entry.

Generalized epilepsy with febrile seizures plus　This is a recently described and common childhood epilepsy syndrome that may show clear autosomal dominant inheritance (Scheffer and Berkovic, 1997). The recognition of this syndrome was a landmark in epilepsy research in that it demonstrated that a single-gene disorder might show very different expression even within the same family. Individual presentations vary, from severe forms such as myoclonic–astatic epilepsy to very mild forms such as a tendency for febrile convulsions beyond the age of 5 years. There are probably several genes responsible for different families with this condition. One family has been shown to have a mutation on chromosome 19q in the gene coding for a voltage-gated sodium channel (*SCN1B*).

Familial temporal lobe epilepsy　This is a fairly common and relatively benign form of epilepsy manifesting as recurrent simple and complex partial seizures (typically *déjà vu*) (*see* Chapter 3).

Familial partial epilepsy with auditory features (linkage to 10q) and **familial partial epilepsy with variable foci** (linkage to 2q) are also seen.

Epilepsy with complex inheritance

These conditions represent the overwhelming majority of epilepsies in which a genetic influence is known or suspected, for example the idiopathic epilepsies of childhood and adolescence. Other diseases resulting from complex disorders of genetic architecture are common in the population and have no clear pattern of inheritance. Conditions with a similar complex (polygenic or multifactorial) inheritance include Alzheimer's disease and multiple sclerosis.

More than one gene, together with environmental factors, influences the development of the disorders. Many susceptibility genes rather than a single disease gene cause most epilepsy syndromes. This has several consequences.

First, individuals with identical phenotypes may have quite different genotypes; for example, some patients with juvenile myoclonic epilepsy show a linkage to chromosome 6p, others one to 15q and others no identified linkage. Second, in some families with the complex trait, there may be few or even only one affected individual, whereas in other families there may be affected individuals scattered in different generations. Third, the phenotype within an affected family may vary considerably such that one individual might have the syndrome of juvenile myoclonic epilepsy while a close relative might have childhood absence epilepsy.

Several major epilepsy syndromes have complex inheritance, their clinical features being described elsewhere:

- febrile seizures
- childhood absence epilepsy
- juvenile myoclonic epilepsy.

Although these are common conditions, large families with the disorders are rare, making linkage studies difficult. Furthermore, genetic and phenotypic heterogeneities increase the problem. There is, however, some evidence to link juvenile myoclonic epilepsy to chromosomes 6p and 15q14, BECTS also to chromosome 15q14, childhood absence epilepsy to chromosome 8q24 and possibly juvenile absence epilepsy to chromosome 21q22.1.

Genetics of epilepsy: conclusion

The genetic basis and molecular mechanism for some epilepsy syndromes have been established. For the large majority of patients with epilepsy, however, and despite suggestions of genetic susceptibility, the genetic basis remains to be identified. It seems likely that a very large number of genetic defects can cause epilepsy. Furthermore, even specific epilepsy syndromes, for example juvenile myoclonic epilepsy, may have several possible genetic causes.

In those human epilepsies in which the molecular basis is understood, the cause appears to be an impairment of function in genes regulating neuronal ion channels, i.e. they are either sodium or potassium channelopathies. Ion channel impairment already explains other paroxysmal neurological disorders, such as periodic ataxia.

Risk of epilepsy in family members

Only rarely, for example in simple Mendelian conditions (*see* above), can the risk to relatives be assessed with any precision, and even here there may be a wide variation in gene expression. In epilepsy as a whole, the risk depends upon several factors:

- the underlying cause
- the number of affected relatives
- the severity of the epilepsy
- the age of epilepsy onset.

In a condition as heterogeneous as epilepsy, guideline figures are very broad and not particularly applicable to any individual case. The risk to other family members is higher in idiopathic generalized epilepsy than in cryptogenic or symptomatic epilepsy. Nevertheless, there is still a surprisingly large genetic predisposition evident in the acquired epilepsies. Asymptomatic EEG abnormalities are found in 20–30 per cent of individuals who have siblings with epilepsy. Table 5.4 provides an idea of the risk to an individual if the named relative has epilepsy (Shorvon, 1995).

Relationship	Percentage risk
Monozygotic twin	70%
Dizygotic twin	10%
Sibling	2–5%
Sibling with seizure onset aged 0–3 years	8%
Sibling with seizure onset aged 4–15 years	4%
Mother	8%
Father	4%
Both parents	25%
Two first-degree relatives	25%
No relative (control)	1.5%

Table 5.4
Overall risk of epilepsy to an individual if the named relative has epilepsy (data from Shorvon, 1995)

The future

Characterizing the molecular basis for inherited epilepsies will allow a more rational classification of epilepsy and offer real hope of providing new methods of diagnosis, as well as of developing and targeting new anti-epileptic treatments (Elmslie and Gardiner, 1995). It may be that a simple blood screen will eventually be able to exclude any one of the hundreds of epilepsy genetic abnormalities that presently await discovery. The availability of such a test, however, might present considerable ethical difficulties concerning consent.

There is an increasing suggestion that many genetically determined epilepsies are 'channelopathies', i.e. associated with disorders of ion flow across membranes. This may have major implications for our understanding of the mechanisms underlying epileptogenesis and for targeting specific treatments.

The management of the epilepsies

Introduction

Epilepsy is not only one of the most common neurological conditions, but also one of the most treatable. In the past few years, the choice of anti-epileptic medication has widened considerably, and the benefit of the newer treatments has become clear. Yet there is much more to the management of epilepsy than the prescription of anti-epileptic medication. Accurate diagnosis and an appreciation of patients' social settings are essential for appropriate and effective management, the emphasis being upon the patient as an individual rather than just upon the symptoms.

When the clinic appointment simply becomes an exercise in counting seizures, juggling with medication and reinforcing restrictions, while seeing a different doctor at each visit, it ceases to be useful. Such situations should be vigorously avoided.

General measures

Apart from driving (for which there is a legal requirement to comply with the regulations), most people with epilepsy ought to be able to lead a fairly normal and fulfilling life. Living with epilepsy inevitably involves living with a degree of risk; it is the doctor's job to point out the risks but not to legislate for their complete avoidance. Restrictions advised by the doctor must balance the risks of potential physical harm to the patient (e.g. from hot saucepans or deep baths) against the risks of psychological damage from the anxiety, social isolation and overprotection that follow such restrictions. The commonsense approach is to point out the hazards of certain situations (e.g. the kitchen, the bath, swimming, cycling, open machinery, carrying a baby on the stairs, climbing trees, apparatus work in the gymnasium) but leave the patient or carer to decide upon any restrictions.

Patient education is an important aspect of effective clinical management. The use of clearly written, unbiased information written specifically for patients is very helpful for them, their families and carers. The provision of information is important in empowering the individual with epilepsy; in general, the more information, the better. For childhood epilepsy, however, an itemization of the features of the relevant syndrome is advised so that the information is as individualized as possible. Some useful sources of patient information about epilepsy are given in the further reading and useful addresses sections (pp. 267 and 269).

Lifestyle measures are covered in Chapter 9.

The first seizure

An admission to hospital may not be necessary following a first seizure, but further investigation is usually required. It is important that patients presenting to the emergency department with a presumed first seizure are referred either to their general pratitioner or to a specialist before considering anti-epileptic medication. In these circumstances, it is helpful to provide patients and their carers with information before their further assessment (Figs 6.1 and 6.2).

Anti-epileptic drug therapy

The large majority of patients with epilepsy will require regular and long-term anti-epileptic medication. A detailed working knowledge of the available medications is essential for clinicians responsible for treating patients with epilepsy.

Figure 6.1
Example of a card to be given to the patient (after Wills and Stevens, 1994)

You have had an epileptic fit.
The doctor has examined you. You do not require admission to hospital.
It is necessary that a responsible adult observes you for 24 hours.
Please rest, take your usual medication and do not drink alcohol.
Arrange to see your family doctor as soon as it is convenient and give him/her the letter describing what has happened to you.
Do not drive until you have discussed the fit with your doctor.

Figure 6.2
Example of a card to be given to the carer (after Wills and Stevens, 1994)

> **Please bring the patient back to the hospital if he or she should:**
> * become increasingly sleepy
> * have another fit
>
> **What to do if another fit occurs**
> Lie the patient down on one side (the recovery position).
> Try to ensure that he/she can breathe easily. This means that the airway must be clear.
> Do not insert objects or fingers into the mouth.
> The fit will usually subside in a few minutes. Stay with the patient. If the attack lasts for many minutes or you feel unable to cope, seek urgent medical help or dial 999 and ask for an ambulance. The ambulance staff will know what to do.

BEFORE STARTING TREATMENT

Four questions must be answered before starting treatment:

1. **Is it epilepsy?** In other words, have there been two or more unprovoked seizures?
2. **Are there provoking factors?** Addressing these might obviate the need for anti-epileptic medication.
3. **Are the attacks sufficiently frequent and troublesome** to justify advising medication?
4. **Does the patient want medication**, even if the doctor advises it?

It is essential to be certain of the diagnosis of epilepsy before anti-epileptic treatment is begun. Anti-epileptic drug treatment implies a firm diagnosis of epilepsy so carries with it important long-term implications for driving, employment opportunity, obtaining a mortgage, life insurance, etc., as well as concerns about long-term treatment being potentially toxic and teratogenic. It is very easy to start medication but much more difficult to withdraw it. Despite pressure, which can often be considerable, upon the physician to 'do something' for the patient with blackouts, there is almost no place for a 'trial' of anti-epileptic medication. If ever such a trial is undertaken, clear end points must be established at the outset. It is particularly unwise to use the EEG as the method of deciding whether or not to start a patient on anti-epileptic medication.

SINGLE SEIZURE

It is not always necessary to start anti-epileptic treatment following a single unprovoked seizure. There are, however, some situations in which it might be reasonable to consider long-term medication.

An **underlying structural lesion** may be suspected, suggested, for example, by a focal seizure onset, abnormal neurological signs or an abnormality on brain imaging.

In **juvenile myoclonic epilepsy**, there is a high likelihood of seizure recurrence, and treatment should be recommended on diagnosis. It must be remembered that the myoclonic jerks of juvenile myoclonic epilepsy are seizure phenomena, and so the convulsion is not really an isolated seizure.

An EEG showing frequent **generalized epileptiform abnormalities** suggests a high likelihood of seizure recurrence.

PRINCIPLES OF ANTI-EPILEPTIC TREATMENT

- **Long term.** Drug treatment for epilepsy is usually long term, often for life, and should therefore be as simple as possible.
- **Single drug.** Start with a single drug; most patients will obtain adequate seizure control and will not experience side effects. Fewer than 30 per cent of patients subsequently require a change of medication or combination therapy (Cockerell *et al.*, 1995).
- The **lowest effective dose** should be aimed for in maintenance therapy.
- **Once or twice daily dosing** is possible and preferred with almost all anti-epileptic medications.
- **Try established treatments first.** The usual initial choices are sodium valproate for any seizure type except neonatal seizures and infantile spasms, and carbamazepine for partial-onset seizures or generalized tonic-clonic seizures. Lamotrigine is also frequently used as an initial mono-therapy.
- The **new drugs** (added to or substituted for conventional drugs), for example gabapentin, lamotrigine, levetiracetam oxcarbazepine, tiagabine and topiramate, all have similar efficacy (Marson *et al.*, 1996) but are generally better tolerated than the conventional drugs.
- **Adverse effects.** Warnings should be given about the dose-related effects and idiosyncratic reactions of medications. Toxicity may result from excessive dosage, low individual tolerance or interactions with other drugs.
- **Persistent or recurrent seizures** may be caused by poor compliance, poor absorption, inadequate dosage or the use of a drug that is inappropriate for that particular patient.
- **Free prescriptions** are available for patients taking anti-epileptic medications in the UK.

ANTI-EPILEPTIC MEDICATION BLOOD LEVELS

For the most part, measuring anti-epileptic blood levels is unnecessary and is much overused in clinical practice. With phenytoin treatment, however, knowledge of levels is essential, especially when establishing the appropriate initial dose or when adding other drugs. Measurement of levels of valproate and of the newer anti-epileptic agents is unnecessary apart from exceptional cases such as overdose, suspected drug-induced encephalopathy, suspected poor compliance or malabsorption.

Indications for anti-epileptic blood level testing

Measurement of phenytoin blood levels is essential, particularly when starting treatment, because the saturation kinetics of phenytoin leave a very narrow therapeutic window between the effective and toxic blood levels; fine adjustment is required to reach the optimal dose.

Young children and learning disabled patients may benefit from drug level estimation since symptoms of toxicity are less reliably obtained.

Suspected overdose, non-compliance or malabsorption may justify blood level measurement, for example with intractable seizures despite the prescription of a high dose of medication.

During **pregnancy**, blood level changes reflect physiological changes but levels of the free drug, as opposed to the protein-bound drug, are little changed; alterations of medication in pregnancy are still best made upon clinical rather than biochemical grounds.

Drawbacks of anti-epileptic blood level testing

A set of numbers generated from the patient's blood can complement, but does not substitute for, a careful history of side effects or of poor compliance. In addition, blood levels are occasionally misleading, as in patients whose 'therapeutic range' (especially of phenytoin) differs from the laboratory 'guidance range'.

Acting upon a blood level alone is potentially harmful, either provoking seizures in hitherto well-controlled patients or denying other patients the chance to try a higher dose for fear of provoking toxicity.

WHICH MEDICATION?

Many anti-epileptic medications are available for prescription; the clinician must choose the treatment or treatments best suited to the individual, taking account of the patient, the epilepsy and the drug itself.

Patient characteristics

Certain characteristics of the patient will help to determine the choice of medication:

- **Age.** The choice of medication will vary when prescribing for differing age groups (infant, child, adult or the elderly). The reasons for this are discussed below.

- **Female.** There are special considerations for prescribing for females owing to potential problems with contraception, fertility, pregnancy, breast feeding, motherhood and possibly bone health (*see* below).
- **Learning disability.** Medications may particularly influence cognitive and behavioural function in patients with learning disability, necessitating a careful selection of medication for this vulnerable group (*see* Chapter 7).
- **Other medical problems.** Underlying medical conditions such as renal or liver disease will influence the type and dose of medication prescribed. Patients on other medications, for example warfarin, are at risk of potentially serious drug interactions.
- **Socioeconomic status.** In underdeveloped countries, the available choice of anti-epileptic medication may be very limited, consequently favouring low-cost preparations such as phenobarbitone.

Epilepsy characteristics

Epilepsy is a heterogeneous condition, and there are many variables that will influence the choice of anti-epileptic medication. Successful treatment depends upon the proper classification of the seizure type and the epilepsy. The neurochemistry of epilepsy, for example the distribution and density of ion channel receptors, differs greatly between individuals, and so it is not surprising that the effectiveness of different treatments also varies widely between patients.

Newly diagnosed versus established epilepsies

In newly diagnosed epilepsy, the aim is for adequate seizure control with the minimum of side effects and inconvenience. Thus, the ideal is to prescribe the lowest effective dose of a medication with as few side effects as possible in a once or twice daily dosage. In established epilepsy, if already controlled, one might be reluctant to change anything unless medication side effects are troublesome; if uncontrolled, each of several medications should be tried in turn.

Idiopathic epilepsies

Idiopathic epilepsy is usually of childhood or teenage onset and responds well, albeit to a limited range of medications, such as valproate, lamotrigine, benzodiazepines, topiramate and phenobarbitone. A few medications may worsen some seizure types: carbamazepine or vigabatrin, for example, can exacerbate absences or myoclonia.

Symptomatic or cryptogenic epilepsies

Almost any of the anti-epileptic medications are potentially effective to some extent in this, the most common form of epilepsy in adults.

Specific epilepsy syndromes

Certain medications are indicated for specific epilepsy syndromes. In West syndrome, the first line of treatment is vigabatrin. Juvenile myoclonic epilepsy and other adolescent-onset idiopathic generalized epilepsy syndromes usually respond to valproate or lamotrigine.

Drug characteristics

A detailed knowledge of anti-epileptic drug characteristics is necessary for best prescribing practice. In selecting anti-epileptic medications, the main aim is to strike the appropriate balance between obtaining drug effectiveness and drug tolerability. An anti-epileptic drug must clearly be effective in controlling seizures. Broadly speaking, all the modern anti-epileptic medications have similar efficacy, at least for partial seizures.

The available anti-epileptic medications show important differences in their tolerability in individual patients. The tolerability of a medication has two aspects:

- **Ease of use.** A drug is easy to use if it can be given once or twice daily, is provided in acceptable formulations and has few interactions.
- **Side effects.** Troublesome side effects, including the risk of teratogenicity, may limit the use of otherwise effective drugs.

Knowledge of drug mechanisms ought to influence the choice of sequences and combinations of medications (*see* below).

Cost is an important but not over-riding factor in prescribing. The costs of various anti-epileptic medications vary widely, the annual costs for an average daily dose in the UK being phenobarbitone £4, phenytoin £40, carbamazepine or valproate £60–120 and the newer drugs £600–1200.

DOSAGE FREQUENCY

Once or twice daily dosing is ideal. Avoid a midday dose if possible since it involves taking tablets to work or school. This is the dose most likely to lead to embarrassment or to be omitted or forgotten.

Carbamazepine in slow-release formulation avoids the need for three times daily administration at higher doses. Gabapentin and higher doses of tiagabine, however, may still require three times daily dosing.

Women planning a pregnancy on medication may be best prescribed their medication three or four times daily in an attempt to lessen the peak serum level that can cross the placenta.

Young children may have to take medication three, or even four, times daily because suitable formulations of slow-release medications may not be available; in addition, their drug half-lives tend to be shorter.

GENERIC OR BRAND NAMES

In patients with epilepsy, it is essential to maintain a constant plasma level of anti-epileptic medications to ensure adequate seizure control. Changes in the formulation of medication may have a critical effect on drug levels in individual patients. Thus, contrary to traditional teaching on medication prescribing, it is safer in patients with epilepsy (where there is a choice of brands) to prescribe anti-epileptic medication by brand name.

RATIONAL PRESCRIBING

Rational prescribing involves making an appropriate choice of medication based upon a knowledge of two factors:

- clinical trials evidence
- mechanisms of drug action.

Clinical trials

Our knowledge of the effectiveness and tolerability of medications derives from data from clinical trials. These, however, have limited aims and several important drawbacks.

Aims of clinical trials

The aims of trials may be regulatory in nature: in order to obtain a licence as an anti-epileptic medication, the preparation must be shown to be more effective than placebo and to have an acceptable level of safety. Trials should also provide clinically useful information about the drug for the prescribing physician.

Drawbacks of clinical trials

- The **artificial situation** is not easily translated into clinical practice.
- Trials are **short term** whereas anti-epileptic medication is usually prescribed for the long term.
- **Resistant epilepsy** is usual among patients recruited to trials, so they do not necessarily represent the epilepsy population. Some patients participate in several clinical trials ('professional patients') and, almost by definition, fail with each new treatment.
- **Extra visits** and patient attention received during a trial can inflate the placebo effect.
- '**Regression to the mean**' occurs. Epilepsy control fluctuates naturally, but patients are more likely to be recruited to a clinical trial if they are going through a bad patch of seizure control and less likely to be recruited if

going through a good patch. Improvement attributable to natural fluctu-ations may account for a significant proportion of the improvement in a short-term trial.

- **Meta-analyses** and comparisons between different trials are difficult to interpret since they involve different epilepsy types, different medication doses and different durations of anti-epileptic medication.
- 'Long-term extensions' (enrichment studies) recruit only those who have already done well on the trial medication; care is therefore required in their interpretation.

Mechanisms of action

The mechanisms of action of most anti-epileptic medications were unknown until relatively recently. This did not limit their clinical usefulness, which implies that a knowledge of mechanisms is relatively unimportant to clinical practice. An understanding of drug mechanisms, however, does allow an attempt at more rational prescribing.

Patients not responding to one drug should perhaps be tried on one with a different known mechanism. Thus, a patient failing on carbamazepine would not next be given lamotrigine or phenytoin since each of these, like carbamazepine, acts primarily upon voltage-dependent sodium channels.

When combining anti-epileptic medications, 'rational polytherapy' would dictate aiming for combinations with different known mechanisms. For example, phenytoin, carbamazepine, phenobarbitone and lamotrigine, each with a similar mechanism, should perhaps not be prescribed in combination.

ONE OR MORE MEDICATIONS

There is surprisingly little trial evidence on which to base the decision of whether to add or substitute anti-epileptic medication. From first principles, however, it would seem better to aim for monotherapy, at least in the first instance, substituting rather than adding drugs if the first drug has failed to control seizures.

HOW TO CHANGE MEDICATION

The conventional way to alter anti-epileptic medication is to add the second drug, build it up to the optimal dose and then withdraw the first drug slowly. There are advantages and disadvantages to this approach. The advantage is that the new drug is already at full dose before the withdrawal of the old drug begins, maintaining best seizure control.

There is, however, the opportunity for troublesome drug interactions and side effects to occur. Also, if the second drug proves immediately effective, the patient and doctor may be reluctant to withdraw the first drug for fear of upsetting the control, thus leaving the patient on two treatments.

The alternative and perhaps preferred approach is to begin the withdrawal of the old drug as soon as the new one is introduced, simultaneously increasing the new and reducing the old one. This might slightly increase the risk of seizures until the new drug has reached its fully effective tissue level, but the patient is more likely to finish on monotherapy.

WITHDRAWAL OF MEDICATION

The decision to withdraw anti-epileptic medication is never easy since patients often have to accept some risk of seizure recurrence during or following withdrawal. There is no right time to withdraw anti-epileptic medication.

In children, a frequent review of the need for anti-epileptic treatment is necessary, and it is reasonable to suggest that withdrawal be considered after 2–3 years of freedom from seizures.

In adults, the issue is often more complicated, and is strongly influenced by considerations of driving and pregnancy. **Driving** is a major reason for continued anti-epileptic medication in adults. Any factor increasing the chance of further seizures will be resisted by people whose livelihood and lifestyle depend upon driving. Furthermore, the UK driving law advises (although it does not require) drivers to refrain from driving from the time of starting anti-epileptic withdrawal until 6 months after the withdrawal is complete.

Pregnancy planning is a major reason for women wishing to withdraw their anti-epileptic medication. No drug is entirely safe in pregnancy, and the ideal is to be off all medications for several weeks before any planned pregnancy. People are often tempted to stop medication on first finding that they are pregnant; unfortunately, most major malformations may already be present at this stage (*see* below).

The prognosis for the successful withdrawal of anti-epileptic medication is best if several of the following factors apply to the patient (MRC, 1991a):

- long duration free of seizures;
- long seizure-free intervals before medication;
- seizure control on only one medication;
- freedom from seizure since starting medication;
- never having had a generalized tonic-clonic seizure;
- idiopathic generalized epilepsy (except juvenile myoclonic epilepsy);
- epilepsies that consistently remit in adolescence, for example benign childhood epilepsy with centrotemporal spikes;
- a normal interictal EEG.

Anti-epileptic medications

Anti-epileptic medications can be broadly grouped into conventional and new drugs:

- **Conventional:** carbamazepine, sodium valproate, phenytoin, phenobarbitone, primidone, benzodiazepines, ethosuximide and acetazolamide.
- **New:** gabapentin, lamotrigine, oxcarbazepine, tiagabine, topiramate and vigabatrin. Summary data for these appear in Table 6.1 (p. 135). Other new agents are levetiracetam and felbamate.

CARBAMAZEPINE

Mechanism and kinetics

Carbamazepine is structurally similar to tricyclic antidepressants and was developed in the 1950s as a mood stabilizer before its anti-epileptic effect was noted. It stabilizes voltage-dependent sodium channels.

Carbamazepine is strongly protein bound, highly lipid soluble and oxidized by the liver's P450 enzyme system into active metabolites including its 10,11-epoxide. It induces the very liver enzymes that metabolize it (autoinduction). After a low starting dose, it is built up to a maintenance dose after several weeks. Its half-life is 5–24 hours while on maintenance treatment.

Indications

Its anti-epileptic effect is limited to partial-onset seizures and generalized tonic-clonic seizures. It may worsen the myoclonic jerks and absences of idiopathic generalized epilepsy.

Dose

- **Adults.** Start at 100 mg twice daily for 7–14 days; maintenance 400–1800 mg per day.
- **Children.** Start at 5 mg/kg per day for 7–14 days; maintenance 10–30 mg/kg per day.

In adults and older children, a slow-release preparation is preferred in order to minimize dose-related side effects and to enable a twice daily prescription even at high doses. Young children who receive carbamazepine in liquid form need thrice daily dosing.

Measurement of blood levels is quite useful and correlates closely with the clinical effect (therapeutic range 20–40 µmol/L or 4–10 µg/mL). In combination with valproate, measurement of total carbamazepine levels can underestimate the amount of carbamazepine metabolites (*see* below).

Side effects

- **Dose-related.** These are common and include tiredness, dizziness and even unsteadiness and double vision.
- **Idiosyncratic.** An allergic rash occurs in about 5 per cent of cases, especially if carbamazepine is introduced rapidly. Rarer complications include neutropenia, inappropriate antidiuretic hormone secretion (giving a low sodium level, which may itself exacerbate epilepsy) and hepatitis.
- **Chronic toxicity.** There are no known serious long-term sequelae from using carbamazepine.
- **Teratogenicity.** Spina bifida (Rosa, 1991) and an excess of other congenital abnormalities (*Lancet*, 1991) are seen in up to 1 per cent of babies exposed to carbamazepine *in utero*. Folate 5 mg daily prior to conception may help to reduce this risk.

Interactions

Effect on other medications
Carbamazepine is a powerful enzyme inducer so affects other medications. Blood levels of warfarin, steroids (including the oral contraceptive pill), lamotrigine, phenytoin and phenobarbitone are all reduced.

Effect of other medications
The blood level of carbamazepine is reduced by phenytoin and phenobarbitone, and increased by erythromycin, cimetidine and dextropropoxyphene (in Distalgesic); care must be taken when prescribing these in combination. Lamotrigine may also elevate the level of carbamazepine metabolites, giving toxic symptoms. Alcohol may interfere with carbamazepine metabolism and so alcohol consumption should be moderated.

Prescribing summary

- Carbamazepine is a first-line treatment for partial-onset and generalized tonic-clonic seizures but is to be avoided in patients with absences or myoclonic seizures.
- Use a slow-release preparation where possible, especially for higher doses.
- Start low and build up to a maintenance (twice daily) dose.
- Blood levels can help in titrating dose but are not essential.
- Warn about rashes, tiredness and interaction with other medications.

- Warn of the need for a higher-dose contraceptive pill and, if the pill was being relied upon for contraception, consider additional methods.
- Restrict alcohol use.
- Hyponatraemia is uncommon, but in elderly patients or those on diuretics, check the electrolyte levels before prescribing (and in the first few weeks of treatment). Should seizures persist in any patient despite carbamazepine, it is worth checking the sodium level.
- Warn about potential teratogenicity (as spina bifida occurs in up to 1 per cent).
- Give with folate 5 mg in women of child-bearing potential who are not taking definite contraceptive measures.
- If given with lamotrigine, toxic symptoms may be caused by an increase in carbamazepine metabolites (and occur despite a therapeutic carbamazepine level) rather than by the lamotrigine itself.

SODIUM VALPROATE

Mechanism and kinetics

Valproic acid was first synthesized in 1881 as an organic chemical solvent. When used with trial anticonvulsants by Berthier Laboratories, the solvent, rather than the (apparently effective) study compounds, was found to be the active agent.

Its mechanism of action is unknown, but possibilities include the raising of gamma-aminobutyric acid (GABA) levels (via inhibited breakdown or increased synthesis) or an action on potassium channels, increasing the hyperpolarization of neurones.

It is well absorbed, strongly protein bound and metabolized in the liver by glucuronidation. Its half-life is 12 hours, but its therapeutic effect lasts longer.

Indications

Valproate has anticonvulsant effects in all seizure types. It is therefore a treatment of choice for idiopathic generalized epilepsies, i.e. most childhood-onset epilepsies, but care is needed in very young children owing to the potential precipitation of hyperammonaemia, with or without associated hepatotoxicity, in this age group.

Dose

- **Adults.** Start at 500 mg daily; the usual maintenance dose is 1000–1500 mg given as a once or twice daily dose.
- **Children.** Start at 10 mg/kg per day; the usual maintenance dose is 20–30 mg/kg per day.

A slow-release formulation is available but is unnecessary for maintaining the anti-epileptic effect, even with once daily dosing. There is a theoretical advantage in women planning pregnancy, in whom the lower peak level (e.g. using a slow-release preparation in divided daily doses) might lessen fetal drug exposure. 'Liquid' rather than 'syrup' preparations are preferred for young children since the former are sugar free.

Measurement of blood levels is unnecessary and unreliable since the proportion of free valproate (and therefore of brain level) varies with different plasma levels.

Side effects

- **Dose-related.** Nausea, vomiting and diarrhoea occasionally occur. In higher doses, tremor, irritability, poor sleep and sometimes confusion may be seen.
- **Idiosyncratic.** Hair loss occasionally happens, the hair sometimes growing back curly. Hyperammonaemia secondary to occult urea cycle disorders and hepatotoxicity is a risk in young children, especially with Alpers' disease (1 in 50 000) but is not a problem in adults.
- **Chronic toxicity.** Weight gain is commonly reported, particularly in young women. Polycystic ovaries appear to be more common in women taking sodium valproate (Isojarvi *et al.*, 1993), perhaps predominantly related to weight gain.
- **Teratogenicity.** Spina bifida occurs in up to 2 per cent of fetuses exposed to valproate. There is recent concern over 'fetal valproate syndrome' and possible developmental delay of children exposed to valproate *in utero* (Adab *et al.*, 2000). Folate 5 mg daily prior to conception may help to reduce this risk.

Interactions

Effect on other medications
Valproate may raise the serum level of other drugs (e.g. lamotrigine, carbamazepine, phenobarbitone and alcohol) by its potent enzyme-inhibiting action, and raise the free level of other medications (e.g. warfarin) by displacing them from protein-binding sites:

- **Lamotrigine.** Great care is required when combining this with valproate; barely half the amount of lamotrigine is needed when given with valproate than when given alone.
- **Carbamazepine.** The inhibition of carbamazepine 10,11-epoxide breakdown can result in a high epoxide level (and thus side effects) despite a 'therapeutic' blood level of carbamazepine.

- **Phenobarbitone.** Sedation, occasionally severe, may occur in combination with valproate owing to an inhibition of phenobarbitone metabolism.
- **Alcohol.** The sedative effect is enhanced by valproate owing to enzyme inhibition.
- **Warfarin.** The anticoagulant effect is enhanced by valproate (the opposite of the effect of enzyme-inducing anti-epileptic medications).

Effect of other medications

The total valproate level is lowered by enzyme-inducing drugs such as carbamazepine and phenytoin. Drugs that displace it from protein-binding sites, for example aspirin, increase the free valproate level.

Prescribing summary

- Valproate is a first-line treatment for generalized seizures.
- It is suitable for all epilepsy types, but care is needed in very young children.
- Build the dose (once or twice daily) to a maintenance level over 2–4 weeks.
- Take care when combining it with lamotrigine.
- Measurement of blood levels is unnecessary.
- Warn about weight gain, tremor, hair loss and polycystic ovaries.
- Warn that alcohol will appear more potent and sedative.
- Warn about the potential for teratogenic spina bifida.
- Prescribe slow-release preparations in divided doses for women planning a pregnancy.
- Give with folate 5 mg in women of child-bearing potential who are not taking definite contraception measures.

PHENYTOIN

Mechanism and kinetics

Phenytoin, a barbiturate-derived hydantoin, was first used as an anti-epileptic in 1938. It stabilizes voltage-dependent sodium channels in a way similar to carbamazepine and lamotrigine.

Phenytoin is strongly protein bound and is metabolized in the liver. The liver enzymes become saturated even at a therapeutic concentration, so a small change in dose may lead to a very large change in plasma level. These notorious 'saturation' kinetics of phenytoin make it difficult to use. There are particular problems when it is used in combination with other enzyme-inducing or protein-bound drugs. The half-life is 13 hours, but this increases with the level of enzyme saturation.

Indications

Phenytoin is indicated for partial-onset and generalized tonic-clonic seizures. The intravenous preparation is rapidly acting and very useful in the treatment of acute symptomatic seizures and status epilepticus.

Dose

- **Adults.** When starting long-term therapy, a loading dose, for example 600 mg daily for 2 days, may be given initially. The usual adult maintenance dose is 300 mg as a single daily dose, adjusted by 25 or 50 mg according to the response, side effects or blood level. In the emergency situation (acute symptomatic seizures or status epilepticus), treatment begins with an intravenous loading dose of 1000 mg given over 20–30 minutes. It is given through a filter and under ECG monitoring. An alternative is fosphenytoin, the pro-drug of phenytoin, which can be given intramuscularly or by intravenous infusion. The monitoring of blood pressure and ECG is still necessary.
- **Children.** The maintenance dose is 3–8 mg/kg per day. Loading is used only in status epilepticus or when the seizures are very frequent; intravenous phenytoin 20 mg/kg is given slowly under ECG control. When given orally to babies, its absorption is impaired if given in close association with milk or formula feeds.

Measurement of blood levels is very useful when using phenytoin because of its difficult kinetics (therapeutic range 40–80 μmol/L ([10–20 μg/mL]).

Side effects

- **Dose-related.** These are common and include unsteadiness, cerebellar ataxia and nystagmus as well as involuntary movements. Mental slowing is often reported with long-term treatment.
- **Idiosyncratic.** There are occasionally rashes and rarely lymphadenopathy.
- **Chronic toxicity.** Cosmetic effects, including coarsening of the facial features, gum hypertrophy, hirsutism and acne, limit its usefulness. Folate and vitamin D deficiency (osteomalacia) are common following long-term use. Cerebellar ataxia and peripheral neuropathy may develop over years and persist despite phenytoin withdrawal.
- **Teratogenicity.** Phenytoin has definite teratogenic potential, the fetal effects including distal phalangeal defects, cleft palate and cardiac defects.

Interactions

Effect on other drugs

Phenytoin is a potent enzyme inducer, lowering the levels of many medications, including carbamazepine and lamotrigine. Blood levels of steroids, including the oral contraceptive pill, are reduced.

Effect of other drugs

Drugs metabolized in the liver (e.g. isoniazid, rifampicin and carbamazepine) interfere with phenytoin's metabolism, tending to increase its blood level. Protein-bound drugs (e.g. aspirin and valproate) displace it from protein-binding sites, thus tending to lower its total level. Enzyme inhibitors (e.g. valproate) increase its blood level. Because valproate has two opposite effects, there is no net change in therapeutic effect.

Prescribing summary

- Use for partial-onset and generalized tonic-clonic seizures but not for absences or myoclonic epilepsy.
- It is very useful in the acute situation, for example status epilepticus.
- Measurement of blood levels is important for monitoring phenytoin dosing.
- Give an initial loading dose and then the (once daily) maintenance dose.
- Make only a small (e.g. 25 mg) change when raising or lowering the maintenance dose.
- Warn about toxic unsteadiness and long-term cosmetic effects.
- Warn of the need for a higher-dose (50 µg oestrogen) contraceptive pill and for additional contraception.
- Take care with interactions when it is used with other medications.
- Restrict alcohol use.
- Warn of potential teratogenicity.
- Give with folate 5 mg to women of child-bearing potential who are not taking definite contraception measures.
- In elderly patients, phenytoin treatment may justify vitamin D supplements and an assessment of mineral bone density.
- In babies, phenytoin is not absorbed from the gut when given in close relationship to milk or formula feeds.

PHENOBARBITONE

Mechanism and kinetics

Phenobarbitone was introduced in 1912 as the first effective anti-epileptic medication. It is much cheaper than other anti-epileptic drugs and still has a major role in developing countries. Owing to its cognitive side effects, however, it now has only a limited role in modern epilepsy management.

It is a barbiturate that enhances GABA transmission and modulates ion channels, thus limiting the spread of an epileptic discharge. It is well absorbed, is 50 per cent protein bound and is metabolized in the liver. It has a long half-life of 60 hours (shorter in children), allowing once daily dosing, but a steady state is not reached for up to 4 weeks after the initial dose.

Indications

Phenobarbitone is effective in partial-onset and generalized seizures. It still has a potential role in the emergency treatment of status epilepticus. It is useful in infants and very young children (if tolerated), since the linear kinetics and well-recognized adverse effects make it easy to manage.

Dose

- **Adults.** 60–180 mg as a single daily dose.
- **Children.** Prescribe up to 8 mg/kg per day in neonates and infants, and 4–6 mg/kg per day in older children.

Measurement of blood levels is occasionally useful, especially if excessive sedation is reported.

Phenobarbitone withdrawal is undertaken only with careful planning and supervision as the risk of rebound seizures is high. Withdrawal must be very slow, for example reducing no faster than 25 per cent every 6 weeks and usually much slower.

Side effects

Phenobarbitone causes changes in behaviour, affect and cognition in up to 50 per cent of patients. In children, hyperactivity (initially) and sleep difficulties can occur.

Being a barbiturate, it produces dependence. Sudden withdrawal may provoke a serious and even life-threatening increase in the number of seizures and psychiatric effects.

Interactions

Effect on other drugs

It is metabolized in the liver and thus interacts with other liver-metabolized drugs, including the contraceptive pill.

Effect of other drugs

Valproate added to phenobarbitone may lead to excess sedation. Alcohol may alter levels of phenobarbitone.

Prescribing summary

- Phenobarbitone is no longer a first-line treatment except in neonates and young infants.
- Prescribe as a once daily dose.
- Warn of possible sedation and cognitive effects.
- Take care regarding interactions, including with the contraceptive pill.
- Restrict alcohol use.
- Withdraw phenobarbitone only slowly.
- Warn of potential teratogenicity and give with folate 5 mg in young women.

PRIMIDONE

Primidone was introduced in 1952. It is a deoxybarbiturate, a pro-drug that is metabolized to phenobarbitone and phenylethylmalonamide in the liver. Its anti-epileptic action is therefore almost identical to that of phenobarbitone. It has no advantage over phenobarbitone as an anti-epileptic yet still has all the disadvantages; it thus has almost no role in modern epilepsy management. Again, there are problems with withdrawal, attempts at which may exacerbate seizures. Therefore a hard core of patients remains on the drug.

BENZODIAZEPINES

Benzodiazepines potentiate GABA receptor activity. They are mild anti-epileptic agents but have a high likelihood of causing sedation, tolerance and withdrawal problems. There are several special indications for benzodiazepines:

- with frequent seizures, when rectal or buccal administration in the home can achieve rapid control;
- the emergency treatment of status epilepticus, with, for example, lorazepam, midazolam or diazepam;
- resistant generalized seizures, such as absences (especially atypical absences) and atonic seizures;
- the short-term treatment of clusters of seizures, for example clobazam in the control of menstrually associated (catamenial) seizures.

ETHOSUXIMIDE

Mechanism and kinetics

Ethosuximide blocks T-calcium channel activation in neurones. It is metabolized in the liver. Its half-life is 20–70 hours, so that once daily dosing is satisfactory.

Indications

The main indication is childhood absence epilepsy, but otherwise resistant myoclonic seizures may respond.

Dose

- **Children.** The maintenance dose is 10–15 mg/kg per day after a slow introduction.
- **Adults.** The maintenance dose is 500–1000 mg per day.

Side effects

- **Dose-related.** Drowsiness, headaches, nausea and abdominal discomfort.
- **Idiosyncratic.** Behavioural effects and, rarely, skin rashes and systemic lupus erythematosus may be seen.

Interactions

There are no significant interactions.

Prescribing summary

- Use as an alternative to valproate for childhood absence epilepsy if no generalized tonic-clonic seizures have occurred.
- Prescribe in a once daily dosage.

OTHER AGENTS

Acetazolamide is a sulphonamide drug that acts as a carbonic anhydrase inhibitor, which can be useful when seizures complicate intermittent ataxias, and for otherwise resistant atonic and atypical absence seizures.

Piracetam is useful in treating myoclonia. Maintenance doses of 20 g daily are usual in adults.

Vitamin B_6 (pyridoxine) is mandatory in pyridoxine dependency. It may be helpful as adjunctive therapy in West and Lennox–Gastaut syndromes. A trial of pyridoxine is worthwhile in all infantile seizures of unknown cause.

Steroids (either adrenocorticotrophic hormone or prednisolone) can be used as short-term therapy for West syndrome since they may eliminate infantile spasms, but other therapies are likely to be needed for continuing seizures. Prednisolone, given as a course, can be effective in some of the epilepsies with cognitive symptomatology, for example Landau–Kleffner syndrome and the syndrome of epilepsy with status epilepticus during slow wave sleep.

Drug	Gabapentin	Lamotrigine	Oxcarbazepine	Tiagabine	Topiramate	Vigabatrin
Mechanism	Unknown site	Sodium channels	Sodium channels	GABA reuptake inhibition	Sodium channels, GABA$_A$ and others	GABA trans-aminase inhibitor
Effectiveness	•	••	••	••	•••	•••
Tolerability	•••	••	••	•	•	•
Spectrum of action	•	•••	•	•	••	•
Few interactions	•••	•	••	•	••	•••

(• = good, •• = very good, ••• = excellent)

Like acetazolamide, **sulthiame** is a sulphonamide and weak inhibitor of carbonic anhydrase. Its anti-epileptic action is only mild, and it is now rarely used.

A **ketogenic diet** is usually reserved for children with very resistant epilepsy syndromes such as severe myoclonic epilepsy and Lennox–Gastaut syndrome. Careful monitoring of the metabolic consequences of the diet is essential.

Immunoglobulins, given intravenously, have been used in both West and Lennox–Gastaut syndromes, but their effects tend to be short lived.

Vitamin E has been suggested for epilepsy but never widely used.

Newer anti-epileptic medications will now be considered, in alphabetical order. With such a wide choice of anti-epileptic medication, it is clearly essential to have a good working knowledge of several treatments. Table 6.1 gives summary data on the commonly used newer medications.

Table 6.1
Newer anti-epileptic drugs: summary data

GABAPENTIN

Mechanism and kinetics

Gabapentin was suggested as an anticonvulsant because of its chemical structure as a GABA analogue. Surprisingly, it does not work through GABA mechanisms but binds to unknown cerebral sites.

It is not protein bound, and 80 per cent is excreted unchanged in the urine. Its half-life is 5–7 hours, hence the need for three times daily dosing to maintain the plasma levels. At very high doses, its absorption is rate limited and the blood level rise is non-linear.

Indications

Gabapentin is a second-line anti-epileptic medication for the treatment of partial-onset seizures. It is ineffective in absence or myoclonic seizures. It has the advantage that it may be introduced rapidly to a maintenance level and, if unsuccessful, can be rapidly withdrawn.

Clinical trials suggest a greater than 50 per cent seizure reduction in about 30 per cent of patients (Marson *et al.*, 1996); with higher doses (up to 3.6 g daily), an increased anti-epileptic effect may be seen.

Dose

- **Adults.** The starting dose is 300 mg daily, increasing rapidly to 1.8 g after 1 or 2 weeks. The manufacturers currently recommend three times daily dosing. If ineffective, it can be withdrawn rapidly without adverse effect.
- **Children.** Those of 6–12 years of age are given 10 mg/kg on day 1, 20 mg/kg on day 2 and then 25–35 mg/kg per day in three divided doses. Maintenance doses are usually 900 mg daily (body weight 37–50 kg).

Measurement of blood levels is not needed.

Side effects

- **Dose-related.** None is expected at the usual doses; at higher doses, common anti-epileptic medication side effects occur, including drowsiness, dizziness, headache and tremor. Overactive behaviour may be observed in children.
- **Idiosyncratic.** None is known, but acute unsteadiness may rarely follow even a small initial dose.
- **Chronic toxicity.** No long-term adverse effects are known.
- **Teratogenicity.** No significant teratogenicity has been found in animal studies, but there are insufficient human data.

Interactions

There are no significant interactions, as expected for a drug that is not protein bound and is excreted unchanged via the kidney.

Prescribing summary

- Use as second-line, add-on treatment for partial-onset seizures.
- Build the dose up quickly (three times daily) to maintenance over 1–2 weeks.
- Higher doses may have a greater anti-epileptic effect.
- Side effects are unlikely.

- There are no significant interactions.
- Measurement of blood levels is unnecessary.
- Its potential teratogenicity in humans is unknown, but animal studies are reassuring.

LAMOTRIGINE

Mechanism and kinetics

Lamotrigine was developed as an anti-folate agent in the belief that folate was an important factor in the genesis of seizures; in fact, lamotrigine is only a weak folate antagonist, and the role of folate in epileptogenesis remains doubtful (Brodie, 1992). Lamotrigine was later thought to be a specific anti-glutamate agent. It is now known to stabilize voltage-dependent sodium channels in a mechanism similar to carbamazepine and phenytoin. Lamotrigine, however, unlike other sodium channel blockers, also appears effective in idiopathic generalized epilepsies, suggesting other, as yet unidentified, mechanisms.

The metabolism of lamotrigine gives difficulty when used in combination with other drugs. It is eliminated by hepatic conjugation, with a half-life of 24 hours in adults.

Indications

Lamotrigine has a broad spectrum of action. It is indicated as a first-line or second-line treatment for partial-onset seizures and generalized tonic-clonic seizures and the atonic seizures of Lennox–Gastaut syndrome, and it also may be effective in generalized absences (particularly atypical absences) and myoclonia. Clinical trials of add-on therapy in partial seizures suggest that about 30 per cent of patients show a greater than 50 per cent reduction in the frequency of seizures (Marson *et al.*, 1996). As monotherapy, its anti-epileptic effect is similar to that of carbamazepine, although it is better tolerated.

Dose

Lamotrigine must be introduced slowly to avoid the development of an allergic rash. Thus, the maintenance level (and therefore its full anti-epileptic effect) is delayed by 4–6 weeks.

The dosing schedule is complicated by its interactions.

- **As monotherapy**, the usual adult starting dose is 25 mg daily, increasing at 2 weeks to 50 mg daily, and further increasing at 4 weeks to 200 mg daily. The usual maintenance dose is 200–400 mg given once or twice daily. In children, the starting dose is 2 mg/kg per day, increasing after 2 weeks to 4 mg/kg per day. When used as monotherapy, doses of about 6–8 mg/kg per day are usual.

- **When adding lamotrigine to valproate**, the recommended adult starting dose is 25 mg on alternate days, increasing at 2 weeks to 25 mg daily, with a usual maintenance dose of 100–150 mg given once or twice daily. In children, the starting dose is 0.15 mg/kg per day or less, with a doubling of the dose at 2-week intervals until there is a therapeutic response or an absolutely maximal dose of 5 mg/kg per day is being given.
- **When adding valproate to lamotrigine**, the dose of lamotrigine must be halved when starting the (adult) valproate dose of 500 mg daily. After 2 weeks, when increasing the valproate to 500 mg twice daily, the lamotrigine may need to be further reduced by 33 per cent.
- **When adding lamotrigine to an enzyme inducer** (carbamazepine, phenytoin or phenobarbitone), the usual adult starting dose is 50 mg daily with a maintenance dose of 300–600 mg given once or twice daily. In children, the dose would start as for monotherapy, but the dose at maintenance may be as high as 10–20 mg/kg per day, particularly if it is used with phenytoin.

Measurement of blood levels is unnecessary since its plasma concentration bears little relationship to its effectiveness.

Side effects

- **Dose-related.** Drowsiness, headache and diplopia are relatively common with increasing dose, especially in combination with carbamazepine, when the effects are caused by carbamazepine metabolites (*see* above).
- **Idiosyncratic.** An allergic rash, sometimes severe in children, is seen in about 10 per cent of cases. It particularly follows rapid introduction or combination with valproate. Severe allergy with Stevens–Johnson syndrome and even fatal liver failure are described in about 1 in 20 000.
- **Chronic toxicity.** A beneficial effect on mood has been reported, but cognition itself appears unaffected.
- **Teratogenicity.** It is not teratogenic in animals, but there are, as yet, insufficient human data.

Interactions

Effect on other drugs
Carbamazepine metabolism is influenced by lamotrigine, giving raised levels of carbamazepine epoxide; thus, in combination, side effects (dizziness and double vision) are common.

Effect of other drugs
Valproate profoundly inhibits lamotrigine's metabolism, so, in combination, only half the usual dose of lamotrigine must be prescribed (*see* above). The combination may have some synergistic anti-epileptic effect.

Prescribing summary

- Use lamotrigine as a first- or second-line treatment for any seizure type.
- Build up the dose (once or twice daily) slowly.
- The dose prescribed depends on other medications taken. Particular care is needed when prescribing with valproate. Bigger doses are needed if it is prescribed with an enzyme inducer.
- Warn about possible rash.
- Measurement of blood levels is unnecessary.
- The potential for teratogenicity is unknown, but folate 5 mg daily is advised for women of child-bearing potential who are not taking definite contraceptive measures.

OXCARBAZEPINE

Mechanism and kinetics

The keto-analogue of carbamazepine was developed as a variant of carbamazepine with fewer side effects. Although there has been widespread experience with it throughout Europe since 1990, it has only recently been licensed in the UK.

It is rapidly absorbed, highly lipid soluble and hydroxylated in the liver (independently of cytochrome P450) to the pharmacologically active 10-monohydroxy-oxcarbazepine. For practical purposes, only the mono-hydroxyl derivative (and no oxcarbazepine) is present in the bloodstream following absorption. Unlike carbamazepine, it does not induce its own metabolism (avoiding the need for a slow introduction) and is not influenced by enzyme-inducing drugs.

The mechanism of action is, like that of carbamazepine, to stabilize voltage-dependent sodium channels.

Indications

Oxcarbazepine is indicated for partial-onset and generalized tonic-clonic seizures. Its effect on myoclonia and absences has not been studied, but it is unlikely to be effective. It is particularly useful when carbamazepine is indicated but poorly tolerated.

Dose

A rough guide is that the maintenance dose is 1.5 times that of carbamazepine. Because there is no enzyme autoinduction, the full dose may be prescribed at the start, though a more gradual introduction is usual.

- **Adult.** The maintenance dose is 600–2400 mg daily as a twice daily dose.
- **Children.** A dose of 15–30 mg/kg per day is appropriate.

Measurement of blood levels may help in planning dose changes.

A switch from carbamazepine to the equivalent dose of oxcarbazepine is possible without a change-over period. In doing so, patients also on liver-metabolized drugs (e.g. phenytoin and lamotrigine) will need a dose reduction as the effect on these drugs of carbamazepine's autoinduction will be lost.

Side effects

Side effects are less troublesome than for carbamazepine:

- **Dose-related.** About 30 per cent of patients experience mild, non-specific, transient symptoms on starting treatment.
- **Idiosyncratic.** Skin rashes are less common than with carbamazepine, making this a good choice for patients responsive to, but allergic to, carbamazepine. About 25–30 per cent of patients allergic to carbamazepine also develop rashes with oxcarbazepine.
- **Chronic toxicity.** Hyponatraemia occasionally occurs, particularly in the elderly; patients also on diuretics should have their sodium level measured before and during the prescription of oxcarbazepine.
- **Teratogenicity.** Despite previous widespread experience, there are still insufficient pregnancy data to be able to specify its risk to the unborn child.

Interactions

Effect on other drugs

The only important interaction is with the oral contraceptive pill. A higher-dose pill (50 µg oestrogen) should be prescribed, and, if relied upon for contraception, additional methods are advised. There is no effect on warfarin.

Effect of other drugs

Unlike those of carbamazepine, oxcarbazepine levels are not influenced by dextropropoxyphene, erythromycin or cimetidine.

Prescribing summary

- This is a first-line treatment for partial-onset seizures and generalized tonic-clonic seizures but is to be avoided in patients with absences or myoclonic seizures.
- It may be useful for patients established on carbamazepine who are experiencing troublesome side effects.
- It is possible to start with a (twice daily) maintenance dose of 600–800 mg daily in adults and 15 mg/kg per day in children. A more gradual starting dose is usually recommended.

- It is possible to switch from carbamazepine to oxcarbazepine without a change-over period. The dose of additional medication such as phenytoin or lamotrigine will need to be reduced.
- Warn of the need for a higher-dose contraceptive pill and for additional contraception.
- Warn about potential teratogenicity (although none has yet been definitely documented).
- Give with folate 5 mg in women of child-bearing potential who are not taking definite contraception measures.

TIAGABINE

Mechanism and kinetics

Tiagabine, like vigabatrin, is a tailor-made anti-epileptic drug that manipulates the inhibitory neurotransmitter GABA. By inhibiting the uptake of GABA into neurones, it raises the GABA level selectively at GABAergic synapses (Leach and Brodie, 1998). Tiagabine has good kinetics, with rapid and complete absorption. It is highly protein bound and metabolized in the liver, with a half-life of 8 hours (although only 3 hours in enzyme-induced patients).

INDICATIONS

Tiagabine is indicated as a second-line, add-on treatment for partial-onset seizures in adolescents and adults. Clinical trials suggest a 50 per cent seizure reduction in up to 40 per cent of patients (Marson *et al.*, 1996). Experience is limited, but it is unlikely to be helpful for generalized absences or myoclonic jerks.

Dose

- **Adults.** The usual dose as add-on treatment is 30 mg daily (in two divided doses taken with food); when combined with enzyme inducers, higher doses (up to 60 mg) and more frequent administration (three times daily) are needed.
- **Children.** Dosing schedules for children have not yet been fully characterized.

Interactions

Effect on other drugs
There are no clinically significant effects on other drugs, including the contraceptive pill.

Effect of other drugs

Enzyme-inducing drugs such as carbamazepine and phenytoin induce a more rapid metabolism of tiagabine, reducing its elimination half-life to 2–3 hours and thereby necessitating three or four times daily dosing.

Side effects

- **Dose-related.** These are fairly common and include dizziness, sedation and headache.
- **Idiosyncratic.** None has been reported.
- **Chronic toxicity.** Despite similarities with vigabatrin, there have been no definite reports of visual field defects attributable to tiagabine.
- **Teratogenicity.** No significant problems have been seen in animal studies, but there are insufficient data to assess its safety in human pregnancy.

Prescribing summary

- Use as an add-on agent for patients with partial-onset seizures.
- Start with 15 mg twice daily (adults) – 20 mg three times daily if combined with enzyme inducers such as carbamazepine or phenytoin.
- Warn about dizziness, sedation and headache.
- Tiagabine does not affect the oral contraceptive pill.

TOPIRAMATE

Mechanism and kinetics

Topiramate has at least four anti-epileptic mechanisms:

1. sodium channel blockade
2. GABA enhancement at the GABA$_A$ receptor
3. AMPA and kainate receptor blockade
4. carbonic anhydrase inhibition.

Topiramate has very good kinetics. It is well absorbed, has low protein binding and is renally excreted. Its half-life is 20–30 hours, making it suitable for once daily administration if preferred.

Indications

Topiramate is indicated as an add-on treatment for intractable partial-onset and generalized tonic-clonic seizures. It brings about a greater than 50 per cent reduction in seizure frequency in about half of patients (Marson *et al.*, 1996). It also appears to be beneficial in generalized epilepsies (Brodie *et al.*, 1998), including those with absences and myoclonus, in which its combination with lamotrigine may be beneficial.

Dose

Topiramate must be introduced slowly, owing to its propensity for sedative and cognitive side effects, particularly in people with neurological handicap or learning disability.

- **Adult.** The usual starting dose is 25 mg on alternate days or once daily, increased at 2-weekly intervals by 25 mg to a usual adult maintenance dose of 100–600 mg given once or twice daily. Occasional patients tolerate 1200 mg daily.
- **Children.** The starting dose is about 1 mg/kg per day, with a gradual increase to a maintenance dose of 3–8 mg/kg per day, although some children will tolerate and respond to higher doses.

Measurement of blood levels is unnecessary as topiramate's effect is independent of the blood level.

Side effects

- **Dose-related.** Cognitive effects are common and include sleepiness, slowed thought and slowed speed of articulation (although not actually dysphasia); these effects often improve with time on the treatment. Psychosis is reported only rarely. Paraesthesiae may occur as a result of its carbonic anhydrase action.
- **Idiosyncratic.** None is known.
- **Chronic toxicity.** Chronic side effects include significant weight loss (a 10–20 per cent loss in 20 per cent of patients). The weight loss may be sufficiently severe to lead to withdrawal of the drug, even if seizures are controlled. There is a 10-fold increased risk of renal calculi, so patients with a history of renal stones should not receive topiramate.
- **Teratogenicity.** The risk is unknown in humans as there are insufficient data, but there is concern from animal studies, in which distal limb abnormalities have been seen following exposure *in utero*. This may, however, be a species-specific effect since other carbonic anhydrase inhibitors, for example acetazolamide, have a similar teratogenicity in rodents but appear safe in humans. The need for a higher-dose oral contraceptive pill with topiramate (*see* below) is nevertheless clearly important.

Interactions

Topiramate has very few interactions.

Effect on other drugs

Topiramate increases oestrogen clearance, so patients taking the oral contraceptive pill require a 50 µg oestrogen preparation and should consider using alternative forms of contraception.

Effect of other drugs

Carbamazepine and phenytoin may lower the topiramate level, but this is rarely of clinical significance.

Prescribing summary

- Use as a second-line treatment for partial and generalized tonic-clonic seizures and possibly for generalized absences and myoclonus. There may be a synergistic effect with lamotrigine in atypical absence and atonic seizures.
- Build up the (once or twice daily) dose only slowly.
- Warn of the possible sedative and ataxic dose-related side effects and of potential weight loss.
- Avoid topiramate if there is a history of renal calculi, and take care if there is a previous psychiatric history.
- Overall, there is little concern over interactions, but women must be warned of the need for a higher-dose oral contraceptive pill.
- Blood levels are unnecessary.
- There is, as yet, insufficient knowledge of its teratogenic effect in humans.

VIGABATRIN

This is an effective anti-epileptic drug, but its widespread prescription has been curtailed since the identification of frequently occurring peripheral visual field defects associated with its use.

Mechanism and kinetics

Vigabatrin was introduced in 1989 as a 'designer drug', being, with tiagabine, one of only two anti-epileptic drugs whose proposed mechanism of action, when developed, proved to be correct.

It is an irreversible (suicidal) inhibitor of GABA transaminase, thus raising GABAs level in the synaptic cleft, enhancing inhibitory transmission. It is rapidly absorbed and excreted largely unchanged.

Indications

Because of its associated visual field problems, the present clinical indications have been considerably curtailed. It is now indicated as an add-on treatment for partial-onset seizures, but only after all other appropriate combinations have proved inadequate. Vigabatrin can worsen some forms of epilepsy, notably myoclonic epilepsies.

It remains, however, the treatment of first choice in West syndrome (infantile spasms), being particularly effective when this is caused by tuberous sclerosis.

Dose

- **Adults.** 500 mg once or twice daily initially, built up over 4–6 weeks to a maintenance dose of 1–3 g daily.
- **Children.** 40–80 mg/kg per day.

Measurement of blood levels is unnecessary, being irrelevant to its cerebral effect.

If vigabatrin needs to be withdrawn, this must be done slowly over at least 2–3 weeks.

Side effects

- **Dose-related.** Sedation, dizziness, headache, unsteadiness and tremor are common. About half of patients gain a little weight. Mild effects on cognition are common.
- **Idiosyncratic.** Vigabatrin may exacerbate myoclonic seizures.
- **Chronic toxicity.** Visual field restriction, often asymptomatic but only rarely reversing after stopping medication, is common (about 40–60 per cent of cases). It occurs between 1 month and several years after starting vigabatrin and is due to the greatly enhanced inhibition of retinal GABA by vigabatrin (Eke *et al.*, 1997).

  There is concentric, predominantly nasal, visual field constriction with temporal sparing (Fig. 6.3). Its severity appears to be related to the cumulative dose (Manuchehri *et al.*, 2000). Patients should be warned to report

Figure 6.3
Vigabatrin-induced visual field constriction. Static threshold perimetry demonstrating a predominantly nasal peripheral field constriction.

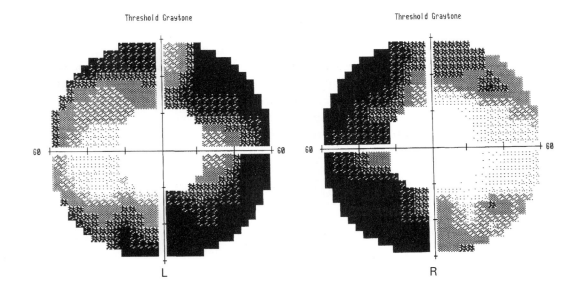

any new visual symptoms that develop after starting vigabatrin treatment. Regular visual field monitoring for patients taking vigabatrin is required. It should be noted that patients treated with vigabatrin who achieve sufficient seizure control to fulfil the epilepsy driving regulations might still be precluded from driving owing to permanent visual field restriction. Visual fields should be quantified before starting treatment, at 6 months and annually thereafter. There are problems interpreting visual field assessments in children under 10 years of age and in the learning disabled.

About 5 per cent of patients develop depression. With a rapid introduction of vigabatrin, this can be severe, occasionally being accompanied by paranoia and psychosis. Children may have extreme behavioural difficulties or occasionally be oversedated.

- **Teratogenicity.** No significant teratogenicity has been reported from animal studies.

Interactions

There are no clinically significant interactions.

Prescribing summary

- Vigabatrin may be used as an add-on treatment for partial-onset and generalized tonic-clonic seizures (but only after other medication possibilities have been shown to be ineffective) and as a first-line treatment in West syndrome.
- Avoid in myoclonic or absence epilepsy.
- Build the dose up over 4–6 weeks (once or twice daily) in adults and over 7–10 days in infants.
- Warn of potential visual field impairment, sedation and depression.
- Avoid in patients with a significant psychiatric history.
- Advise patients to report any new visual symptoms promptly.
- Monitor the visual fields using static perimetry before treatment, at 6 months and then annually. Withdraw vigabatrin if significant field loss develops.
- Measurement of blood levels is unnecessary.
- There is no concern over interactions.
- Withdraw vigabatrin only slowly.
- The teratogenicity potential is unknown.

LEVETIRACETAM

Levetiracetam is a potent anticonvulsant with few interactions and has so far shown a favourable safety and side effect profile. The mode of action is unknown but appears unique. There are no major drug interactions and, in particular, no interaction with the pill or warfarin. There is hope that levetiracetam may have a broad spectrum of action including not only partial-onset and secondary generalized seizures, but also effects on myoclonia, absences and photosensitivity.

If the promise from the clinical trials is maintained in clinical practice, levetiracetam is likely to be an important addition to the current range of anti-epileptic medications (Shorvon, 2000).

FELBAMATE

This is an effective anti-epileptic drug for partial seizures and for seizures associated with loss of posture in the Lennox–Gastaut syndrome. Its use has, however, been curtailed because of rare but occasionally fatal (one in 4000 patients) bone marrow and hepatic side effects (Dichter and Brodie, 1996).

Felbamate has multiple mechanisms, including an effect on sodium channels, enhancing GABA and blocking NMDA receptors.

Felbamate's drug interactions make it difficult to use, and there is a need for regular blood tests of leukocyte count and liver function tests.

ANTI-EPILEPTIC DRUGS ON THE HORIZON

Despite the range of new anti-epileptic drugs and advances in the surgical management of epilepsy, there remains a clear need for newer anti-epileptic medications. Several drugs are currently under consideration and may be marketed in the near future.

Remacemide

Remacemide, a pro-drug, is metabolized to a biologically active metabolite. Initial studies of remacemide as an add-on treatment were encouraging, but a meta-analysis of the available placebo-controlled studies has shown only limited efficacy (Leach *et al.*, 1999). It has important interactions with enzyme-inducing anti-epileptic medications such as carbamazepine and phenytoin. It is generally well tolerated at therapeutic doses.

Zonisamide

Zonisamide is a sulphonamide analogue already available in Japan. It shows anti-epileptic effect in many seizure types including partial and secondary generalized seizures, primary generalized seizures (although its effect on absences and myoclonic seizures remains unclear) and West syndrome. The recommended starting dose in adults is 100–200 mg daily, titrated to 200–400 mg daily. At higher doses, plasma level monitoring is advisable because of enzyme saturation. Enzyme-inducing drugs such as carbamazepine and phenytoin speed up its elimination. Overall, zonisamide appears reasonably well tolerated, although there are reports of occasional idiosyncratic reactions including Stevens–Johnson syndrome, agranulocytosis and renal stones.

Losigamone

Losigamone is a novel anticonvulsant compound with anxiolytic and antidepressant properties. It has a short half-life of about 4 hours, thus requiring a 3–4 times daily dosing regimen. Its metabolism is stimulated by carbamazepine and phenytoin. Preliminary placebo-controlled add-on data in refractory epilepsy suggest that losigamone is effective in reducing seizure frequency. It is generally well tolerated.

Other promising anti-epileptic compounds include pregabalin, rufinamide, retigabine, soretilide and dezinamide (Davies and Smith, 2000).

Epilepsy surgery

Surgery is no longer considered a last resort in epilepsy management. Selected patients with localization-related epilepsy, particularly children and teenagers, can obtain major benefit and often freedom from seizures after surgery.

ADVANTAGES OF EPILEPSY SURGERY

Successful surgery leads to effective seizure control, which has obvious advantages:

- Effective seizure control can dramatically improve a patient's quality of life. If surgery is performed when the patient is a child or teenager, seizure control may avoid the development of the major handicaps and stigma that commonly accompany a diagnosis of epilepsy.
- Long-term anti-epileptic medications may not be necessary.
- The risk of sudden death associated with epilepsy is minimized.

DISADVANTAGES OF EPILEPSY SURGERY

- **Mortality.** The operative mortality is very low, perhaps about 0.5 per cent. This must be put into context of the mortality of having seizures. A major justification for epilepsy surgery is the concern about sudden death in epilepsy since this has an incidence of 1 per 100 per year in medically intractable epilepsy.
- **Morbidity.** Patients undergoing temporal lobectomy frequently develop

a visual field deficit (homonymous upper quadrantanopia), which is significant in about 10 per cent of cases. This may preclude legally holding a driving licence should the patient subsequently become seizure free. Other significant problems are the risk to speech and memory.

- **Social factors.** Some patients find paradoxical difficulty adjusting to being seizure free. New responsibilities and expectations present a considerable emotional burden to someone who has known only a dependent lifestyle.

SURGERY AND THE EPILEPTIC FOCUS

Successful surgery requires the identification of both components of the epileptic focus: the epileptogenic lesion and the epileptogenic zone.

- **The epileptogenic lesion.** This is the structural lesion on imaging that is associated with the development of seizures.
- **The epileptogenic zone.** This is the area of seizure onset and propagation; it is the site of seizure origin on an ictal EEG and the area the surgeon aims to resect.

The ideal operative strategy is to resect the epileptogenic lesion with the surrounding cortex that contains the epileptogenic zone. Identifying the epileptogenic lesion is usually easy, but identifying the epileptogenic zone is more difficult because the available information may be misleading.

There may be **misleading symptoms**. The symptoms of a seizure may develop at a distance from the epileptogenic zone (symptomatogenic zone), giving falsely localizing information. Temporal lobe seizures, for example, may derive from a frontal lobe lesion.

Misleading imaging may occur. The site of the epileptogenic zone is not necessarily within the visible lesion (e.g. in polymicrogyria) and so cannot be determined from imaging alone. Even if an identified lesion is closely associated with the seizure origin, the epileptogenic zone often extends into the surrounding cortex. Conversely, in very large lesions, the epileptogenic zone may occupy only a small area of the lesion.

A **misleading EEG** may be recorded. A surface EEG may give misleading information because it identifies only that part of the cerebral cortex which is involved in the seizure, and not necessarily the site of seizure origin.

There is no short cut to identifying the epileptogenic zone. The problem is greater with lesions with indistinct boundaries (such as cortical dysplasias) than with more clearly demarcated lesions (such as benign tumours).

For best surgical results, the history, EEG and imaging must all point to one area, i.e. all test results must 'line up'.

PATIENT SELECTION

Patients selected for epilepsy surgery will have as many as possible of the following characteristics:

- **young age**, a clear advantage in undergoing epilepsy surgery. Teenagers are particularly suitable, since they are old enough to participate in the decision-making process yet still young enough to have avoided the major (and potentially permanent) social handicaps associated with epilepsy;
- **partial-onset and/or secondary generalized seizures** (localization-related epilepsy), usually of temporal lobe origin;
- **seizures resistant to anti-epileptic medication**, for example failure of three appropriate anti-epileptic medications, each at a maximum tolerated dose for a minimum of 6 months with adequate compliance;
- **certainty of the site of seizure origin** (the epileptogenic zone);
- an **excellent concordance** between clinical features, radiological findings and neurophysiology;
- a **minimal risk to memory and speech** in temporal lobe epilepsy, and to limb function in frontoparietal epilepsy, if the epileptogenic zone were resected.

PRE-OPERATIVE EVALUATION

The surgery itself is the most straightforward part of the procedure. The major problem is ascertainment that the correct piece of brain is being removed, without undue danger to essential functions, especially memory and speech. Only about a third of patients considered for surgery pass the rigorous selection procedure.

Preconditions for epilepsy surgery

- **Diagnostic certainty.** The history and witness account must leave no doubt that the patient is experiencing epileptic seizures and that these are of partial-onset (including secondary generalized) rather than primarily generalized.
- **Medication-resistant seizures.** The patient's seizures must be disabling despite adequate medication(s).
- **General health.** There must be no medical contraindication to surgery.
- **Degenerative or metabolic disease.** This must not be the cause of the epilepsy.

Identifying the epileptogenic zone

Electroencephalogram
Interictal recordings can be misleading, for example normal or with bilateral abnormalities, so ictal monitoring is essential. Ictal monitoring involves

recording the surface and depth EEG (e.g. using foramen ovale leads for temporal lobe surgery) with video over several days. The anti-epileptic medication is reduced or stopped in order to capture typical attacks. Ictal recordings must leave no doubt that the seizures arise consistently from one epileptogenic focus.

Structural imaging

Computed tomography brain scanning is inadequate for epilepsy surgery evaluation. High-resolution magnetic resonancy imaging (MRI) brain scanning is necessary to demonstrate subtle lesions responsible for recurrent partial seizures. MR scans performed on older and less powerful machines, or to non-standard protocols, may miss relevant lesions. Thus, a normal MR scan does not necessarily preclude surgery.

In order to proceed to epilepsy surgery, a structural lesion must usually have been demonstrated at the site of the epileptogenic focus on ictal EEG. This might, for example, be mesial temporal sclerosis, a tumour, a cavernoma or heterotopic grey matter. An abnormally small hippocampus without sclerosis may be considered a sufficient abnormality. Epilepsy surgery is unlikely to be successful if a high-resolution MR brain scan is normal.

Functional imaging

Interictal single photon emission computed tomography (SPECT) or positron emission tomography (PET) scanning may demonstrate focal hypometabolism in the epileptogenic focus. Ictal SPECT may show hypermetabolism at the same site. Functional MRI is becoming increasingly useful in evaluating patients for epilepsy surgery. Functional imaging is particularly useful when the MR scan is normal. It also helps when MRI shows a large (and unresectable) lesion but the epileptogenic focus might be shown to occupy only a small part of this. Functional imaging may be particularly helpful in planning surgery for malformations of cortical development as the epileptogenic zone is often outside the area of visible abnormality.

Safety of memory and speech function

Wada testing

During an intra-arterial angiogram, and with the patient awake, sodium amytal is injected into each carotid artery and thus reaches each hemisphere in turn. With each side anaesthetized, a brief assessment of psychological function, speech and memory is made. This gives certainty of language laterality and helps to determine the risk of memory loss following medial temporal resection. Selective Wada procedures, for example selectively canalizing the posterior cerebral artery, a procedure associated with a higher risk to the patient, may be needed in patients who unexpectedly fail a Wada test.

Functional MRI

This imaging is based upon the different magnetic characteristics of oxygenated and deoxygenated blood and seems likely eventually to replace Wada testing by non-invasively demonstrating the anatomical location of speech and specific memory functions.

EPILEPSY SURGERY PROCEDURES

Lesional

This refers to epilepsy surgery in which there is a demonstrated lesion closely associated with the epileptogenic zone.

- **Temporal lobectomy** is the most effective and therefore the most common surgical procedure for epilepsy, particularly for mesial temporal sclerosis. Extensive resections do not necessarily give a greater chance of seizure freedom, and so more limited procedures, for example selective amygdalohippocampectomy, are preferred. Overall, 50–70 per cent of the patients selected for temporal lobe surgery become seizure free, 20–25 per cent significantly improve and 10–15 per cent obtain no worthwhile improvement (Lamoureux and Spencer, 1995).
- **Frontal lobectomy**, tailored to the epileptogenic focus, is the second most common focal resection. The success rate is lower than for the temporal lobe, particularly if there is no demonstrable structural lesion. Overall, 30–50 per cent of these patients who are selected for surgery become seizure free, 20–40 per cent are markedly improved but 25–35 per cent are no different.

The results of lesional epilepsy surgery for well-defined focal lesions such as mesial temporal sclerosis, ganglioglioma, etc., are generally very good (up to 80 per cent seizure free at 2 years). Patients with cortical dysplasia as the cause of their epilepsy do less well (less than 50 per cent seizure free at 2 years) since the lesion is often not truly focal at a microscopic level (Sisodiya, 2000); functional imaging and electrocorticography are helpful in deciding on surgery in these cases.

Non-lesional

This refers to epilepsy surgery in which the epileptogenic zone is widespread or lies within unresectable cortex, for example in the primary motor area. Here, surgery aims to limit the seizure discharge from spreading. Suitable candidates might be young patients with symptomatic generalized epilepsies such as Lennox–Gastaut syndrome.

Corpus callostomy

Corpus callosotomy is a palliative procedure aimed at limiting the bilateral spread of intractable generalized seizures, particularly atonic seizures in which the patient falls. It is usually reserved for patients severely disabled by epilepsy and with multiple seizure types; patients often have other neurological impairments. It is unlikely to eliminate all seizures in all patients but may improve safety and quality of life for the patient and carers.

Hemispherectomy

Hemispherectomy can be very effective in children with a prenatal or perinatal onset of hemiplegia and refractory seizures. A possible reduction in hand function and the acquisition of a visual field defect are usually well compensated for by very useful seizure control.

Multiple subpial transections

Multiple subpial transection involves making many tiny cortex-deep cuts, respecting the blood vessels, to isolate blocks of cortex by interfering with horizontal transmission within the cortex. This procedure has been used particularly in the Landau–Kleffner syndrome. Long-term follow-up data are awaited.

'GAMMA KNIFE' SURGERY (RADIO SURGERY)

'Gamma knife' surgery has become possible with advances in radiotherapy, computing and imaging techniques. It is particularly used as an alternative to surgery in treating arteriovenous malformations but has been applied to the treatment of small tumours and metastases, and, more recently, as an alternative to temporal lobe resection for mesial temporal sclerosis.

The technique relies upon an accurate localization of the target area by computed imaging. A frame is fixed to the patient's skull, and MR scanning precisely maps the lesion. The computer is programmed to reveal some of the 200 separate sources of ^{60}cobalt around the patient's head (focusing radiation on the target lesion) for a predetermined time. After the treatment, the patient is able to go home with no special precautions. The benefit of the radiotherapy then follows over several months, with shrinkage and sometimes disappearance of the target lesion.

Although there has been a wide experience of radio surgery worldwide, there are surprisingly few randomized controlled trials or detailed studies of long-term benefit or safety. Nevertheless, the technique is fast becoming the surgical treatment of first choice for small arteriovenous malformations to prevent the risk of bleeding. Its use in the treatment of mesial temporal sclerosis is so far only anecdotal and not widely practised.

Non-drug treatments of epilepsy

STRESS CONTROL

Stress, resulting from seizures or the threat of seizures, may affect epilepsy in several ways:

- hyperventilation, lowering the seizure threshold or mimicking seizures;
- increased alcohol consumption;
- impaired sleep quality.

Relaxation techniques (meditation, aromatherapy and yoga) are often surprisingly effective in improving seizure control and can be recommended to anyone with poorly controlled epilepsy.

DIET

A ketogenic diet can be helpful in otherwise poorly controlled childhood epilepsy. It is unpleasant for the child and family, occasionally has serious complications (Ballaban-Gil *et al.*, 1998) and is now rarely used.

VAGUS NERVE STIMULATION

This is a novel and invasive treatment for patients with resistant, long-standing partial-onset epilepsy (Schachter and Saper, 1998). The mechanism of action is unknown but it is based upon the knowledge that EEG rhythms in animals can be influenced by vagus nerve stimulation. The technique involves the intermittent stimulation of the left vagus nerve by a programmable signal generator implanted in the chest cavity. The left vagus is chosen because it has more afferent fibres than the right, as well as because it innervates the cardiac ventricles more than the atria: stimulation here is less likely to lead to cardiac rhythm disturbances.

The effectiveness of vagus nerve stimulation is difficult to assess because of the confounding placebo effect of undergoing a surgical procedure and then experiencing the tingling sensation and hoarse voice associated with the intermittent electrode stimulation. Trials using high-versus-low dose stimulation do appear to show a benefit (Handforth *et al.*, 1998), and there have been occasional notable successes. Overall, vagus nerve stimulation is about as effective as adding a new anticonvulsant (30–50 per cent of patients obtain a greater than 50 per cent seizure reduction) but has the real advantages of 100 per cent compliance with treatment and no drug interactions or medication side effects. The method appears to be safe and well tolerated, the main side effects being pain around the implantation site, hoarseness and swallowing problems.

Acute treatment of seizures

Seizures usually occur as isolated, infrequent events or as frank status epilepticus. Rarely, the onset of epilepsy is explosive, with very frequent recurring seizures. For generalized tonic-clonic seizures, loading with phenobarbitone or phenytoin (as for status) may be appropriate while the longer-term therapy, for example valproate, is introduced. For brief, frequent partial seizures, carbamazepine, with its short half-life, may be the best option. When other types of seizure present acutely, oral benzodiazepines (diazepam or clonazepam) may give short-term relief. If the seizures are sufficiently frequent to interfere with swallowing, treatment as for status epilepticus should be instituted.

Status epilepticus

This is an important and life-threatening condition (Shorvon, 1994) and can be divided into two broad categories:

- convulsive (tonic-clonic)
- non-convulsive.

The spectrum of status epilepticus is somewhat wider in children than in adults and includes neonatal status, febrile status epilepticus and electrical status confined to slow wave sleep. However, the concept of convulsive and non-convulsive forms remains useful.

CONVULSIVE (TONIC-CLONIC) STATUS EPILEPTICUS

This is the more common and clinically more significant form.

Definition
A practical definition is:

> Tonic-clonic seizures persisting for more than 30 minutes without recovery of consciousness between them.

Some clinicians advise 5 minutes of continuous seizures in the definition, reflecting an increased awareness of the need for urgent intervention to prevent seizure-induced neurological damage.

Incidence

Using the '30 minute' definition, status epilepticus is uncommon in the developed world. Seizures lasting for more than 5 minutes, however, occur in 5 per cent of patients with epilepsy and account for 0.1 per cent of all visits to emergency departments. Status epilepticus is most common in children and the elderly, reflecting the common underlying causes. About half of patients with status epilepticus have no previous history of epilepsy.

Aetiology

- **Fever.** Status epilepticus may arise *de novo* in febrile children, particularly with viral encephalitic illnesses.
- **Pre-existing epilepsy.** An important cause of status epilepticus is a loss of control of pre-existing epilepsy, associated most often with poor treatment compliance but sometimes with intercurrent illness.
- **Structural brain lesion.** Stroke, tumour and head injury are the most important causes of status epilepticus in adults, which may even be their presenting symptom.
- **Metabolic changes.** Alcohol and drug withdrawal are important causes of status epilepticus in adults. In neonates, hypoxic–ischaemic encephalopathy is most likely, but hypoglycaemia, hypocalcaemia, hypomagnesaemia, hyperammonaemia and pyridoxine dependency should be considered.

Pathophysiology

Early

- **Lactic acidosis.** Continuous seizures increase the brain's demand for blood, oxygen and glucose; lactic acidosis results when demand outstrips supply.
- **Increased adrenergic output.** Tachycardia and hypertension, already provoked by continuous seizure activity, increase further with lactic acidosis.
- **Cerebral oedema.** This is caused by the combination of hypoxia and lactic acidosis. Systemic hypertension further raises the intracranial pressure.

Late

Cerebral hypoxia results from several mechanisms:

- **Cerebral autoregulation** becomes disturbed as status epilepticus becomes established.
- **Hypotension and respiratory depression** may be caused by anti-epileptic medications, especially benzodiazepines.

- **Cardiac arrhythmias** may result from the metabolic upset, the cardiac effects of medication and the seizures themselves.
- **Cerebral oxygen demand** increases during seizures.
- **Cerebral blood flow** falls as a result of raised intracranial pressure during seizures.
- **Excitotoxic amino acids**, for example glutamate and aspartate, may cause direct neuronal damage.

Management

General points

- Once repeated tonic-clonic seizures occur, they must be treated quickly and aggressively.
- Treatment aims to prevent the development of status epilepticus, so the emergency treatment of repeated seizures begins at 5 minutes.
- Investigations to determine the aetiology of seizures are appropriate when time permits, but treatment must not be delayed while awaiting investigations or results. The blood glucose level should be determined immediately in all cases. Patients should not be sent for brain scans etc. whilst actually convulsing as brain damage may result from seizures prolonged beyond 30 minutes.
- Status epilepticus is best managed on an intensive care unit.
- Ask yourself whether these are really seizures. 'Status pseudoepilepticus', a manifestation of non-epileptic attack disorder, is almost as common as status epilepticus in adults presenting with apparently resistant seizures (*see* Chapter 7).

Immediate

In the emergency situation, there are several imperatives:
- Establish an airway and ventilation, and assess vital signs.
- Ensure adequate circulation and exclude severe hypotension.
- Rapidly determine the blood glucose level and take blood for biochemistry, toxicology and anti-epileptic drug levels.
- Consider giving thiamine 100 mg (if alcoholism is suspected) and 50 per cent glucose intravenously (if hypoglycaemia is identified).

2–4 minutes

A benzodiazepine is the treatment of first choice. Benzodiazepines act rapidly but, being lipophilic, can accumulate and cause respiratory depression. Lorazepam is better than diazepam because it has a longer action and, being less lipid soluble and entering the brain more slowly, can be given more rapidly, is longer acting and less cumulative, and carries much less risk of hypotension and hypoventilation.

- The preferred regimen is lorazepam, diluted to 50 per cent in an intravenous infusion, given at 0.1 mg/kg and repeated after 2 minutes if the seizures continue.
- If intravenous access is not obtained readily, rectal diazepam in solution 0.5 mg/kg for children should be given. The maximum initial dose is 10 mg.
- An alternative for treating outside hospital (e.g. in a hostel or school) is to give midazolam 0.2–0.4 mg/kg either nasally or buccally (between the cheek and teeth) (Scott *et al.*, 1999).

5 minutes

If the seizures do not respond to a benzodiazepine after 5 minutes, a rapidly acting second-line treatment is required. Traditionally, phenytoin is given as an intravenous loading dose (15–20 mg/kg over 20–30 minutes, e.g 1200 mg over 25 minutes in an adult). Phenytoin in solution is very irritant and must be given by slow infusion. It can lead to hypotension and cardiac arrhythmias so a cardiac monitor must be running during an infusion. Fosphenytoin, the pro-drug of phenytoin, is converted to phenytoin with a half-life of 15 minutes. Although it is more expensive than phenytoin, it can be given more rapidly and is better tolerated; it may soon replace phenytoin in this role, although ECG and blood pressure monitoring remain essential.

- The preferred regimen is fosphenytoin (expressed as phenytoin equivalents) 20 mg/kg infused at 150 mg per minute (e.g. 1200 mg over 8 minutes in an adult).

25 minutes

If the seizures prove resistant to both lorazepam and phenytoin (or fosphenytoin), i.e. 30–40 minutes into treatment, the question again should be asked whether these are non-epileptic seizures. If further treatment is needed, the patient will need to be managed on an intensive care unit in order to allow administration of more powerful and sedative medications.

- The recommended treatment at this stage is a loading dose of phenobarbitone 10 mg/kg given intravenously at a rate of 100 mg per minute (e.g. 700 mg over 7 minutes in an adult).

40 minutes (ventilator stage)

If the seizures persist, and they are definitely seizures, there is no option but to intubate and ventilate the patient. There is no consensus on the anaesthetic to be used, the choice being between thiopentone, propofol (a short-acting $GABA_A$ agonist) and midazolam (a short-acting benzodiazepine). Thiopentone and midazolam are anti-epileptic but have problems of accumulation, potentially leading to later difficulties with withdrawal. Propofol is not anticonvulsant (and may even be proconvulsant) but is not as cumulative.

The purpose of anaesthesia is not just to prevent the tonic-clonic convulsions but, more importantly, to stop the damaging seizure activity in the brain. It is therefore essential that anaesthetic (rather than just sedative) doses are used and the EEG is continuously monitored. The target is to suppress the brain rhythms to the point of 'burst suppression' on EEG. The patient should then be woken every 2–4 hours to check whether the seizures have stopped. Pulmonary artery wedge pressure monitoring is helpful in determining fluid balance needs.

- If the seizures persist, and they really are seizures, the patient must be ventilated.

Underlying cause

Excluding 'status pseudoepilepticus'
A very common problem is the misdiagnosis of psychogenic non-epileptic status (status pseudoepilepticus); too often this results in intubation, ventilation and other assaults on someone whose problem is behavioural rather than epileptic. It accounts for as many as half of all adult emergency admissions with a diagnosis of status epilepticus (Howell *et al.*, 1989) but rather less with children. True status epilepticus is rare in young, otherwise healthy, adults. Suspicion should be aroused if the person in status epilepticus is a young woman (it is eight times more common in women than men) in whom there is normal intelligence, no neurological deficit or brain scan abnormality and extensive hospital case notes from previous consultations and admissions (*see* Chapter 7).

Determining the cause
Further investigations may be needed to determine the underlying cause. Infections such as encephalitis and cerebral abscess are examples of progressive intracranial causes of status epilepticus for which cerebral imaging (and, for encephalitis, lumbar puncture) may be appropriate. Metabolic causes and drug withdrawal, particularly sudden non-compliance, need to be considered.

Preventing recurrence
While instituting emergency treatment, some maintenance therapy is needed to prevent seizure recurrence. The choice of treatment will depend on the

cause of the status. If the patient is already on anti-epileptic medication (and the status epilepticus has possibly resulted from poor compliance), his or her previous medication needs to be restarted, by nasogastric tube if necessary. For newly diagnosed epilepsy presenting as status epilepticus there is a high probability of later seizure recurrence and so some maintenance treatment may be needed. In the short term, it may be wise to use maintenance phenytoin or phenobarbitone while deciding on the optimal choice for long-term therapy.

Treating complications

Certain important complications of established status epilepticus, for example rhabdomyolysis, hyperthermia, renal failure and cerebral oedema, may require specific treatment.

Role of the EEG

If seizures are quickly controlled following emergency measures, EEG monitoring may not be necessary. Such monitoring becomes increasingly important in the management of advancing stages of status epilepticus. In the 'ventilator' stage, it is essential to monitor the EEG and aim for the suppression of electrical seizure activity. In contrast, an EEG showing only movement artefacts during episodes, and normal rhythms between convulsions, strongly indicates a non-epileptic attack disorder.

Prognosis

Status epilepticus is a serious condition with a significant mortality (5–10 per cent) and morbidity, up to 30 per cent in children and the elderly:

- In **adults**, the mortality often directly relates to the aetiology. Thus, 90 per cent of adult deaths from status epilepticus result from the underlying stroke, encephalitis, tumour or trauma. Long-duration status epilepticus and the presence of hypoxic/metabolic complications reflect the aetiology and are poor prognostic factors. The best outcomes are seen in those with a previous history of epilepsy whose status epilepticus has arisen through poor compliance.
- In **infants and children**, the developing brain is more vulnerable to damage from seizures and so the prognosis is determined by the severity and duration of the seizures themselves.

Epilepsia partialis continua

This is an uncommon condition manifesting as resistant, simple, partial seizures. A typical manifestation may be the persistent involuntary jerking of one side of the body without altered consciousness.

The condition may be of **adult onset**. In adults, especially the elderly, it is most usual in relation to cerebrovascular disease. There are often paroxysmal lateralizing epileptiform discharges on the EEG. The condition is notoriously resistant to treatment, and there is a real danger of doing the patient more harm than good by aggressive management. It is often self-limiting so it may be better to await remission rather than risk suppressing the conscious level with large doses of anti-epileptic medication.

Rasmussen encephalitis occurs in young children and is characterized by epilepsia partialis continua with an associated progressively acquired hemiparesis. Pathologically, chronic, patchy severe encephalitis is seen. There is a poor response to anti-epileptic drugs, and hemispherectomy may be necessary.

Herpes simplex encephalitis often first manifests as well-localized epilepsia partialis continua for some hours or a day or two before reduced consciousness and other signs of encephalitis become evident.

NON-CONVULSIVE STATUS

This is less common and comprises three major forms:

- complex partial status epilepticus (more common in adults);
- absence, or atypical absence, status epilepticus (more common in children);
- electrical status epilepticus during slow wave sleep.

Complex partial status epilepticus

Aetiology
Complex partial status epilepticus usually occurs against a background of previous epilepsy. It may be triggered by infection, alcohol, drugs or electroconvulsive therapy.

Clinical features
It presents as periods of confusion lasting for hours or even weeks or months. There are occasionally motor features such as myoclonic jerks or automatisms.

Investigations
Complex partial status epilepticus is the major indication for obtaining an EEG in a confused patient. The EEG shows frequent or continuous spiking or spike-and-wave activity.

Management
Treatment is difficult as the condition is often relatively resistant to standard anti-epileptic medications. It is important to strike an appropriate balance

between aggressive attempts to control seizures and the avoidance of unnecessary sedation and other medication side effects. Although benzodiazepines are often effective in the short term, the control of seizures by non-sedating medications, and the avoidance of anaesthesia, is preferred.

Prognosis
The outlook for patients with complex partial status epilepticus is surprisingly poor and related to the underlying cause. There is a high likelihood of recurrence, even after successful initial seizure control.

Absence status epilepticus
It is important to distinguish this (childhood) condition from complex partial status. There are four types (Shorvon, 1994).

Typical absence status epilepticus
This condition arises in about 5 per cent of patients with childhood absence epilepsy and manifests as a clouding of consciousness. Emergency treatment is with intravenous benzodiazepines such as diazepam or lorazepam. Plans for longer-term treatment include the initiation of valproate or ethosuximide (or lamotrigine) therapy. The prognosis is good.

Atypical absence status epilepticus
This condition arises in patients with symptomatic generalized epilepsies, for example Lennox–Gastaut syndrome. It may respond poorly to benzodiazepines, although these remain the first-choice treatment. Paraldehyde and intravenous chlormethiazole are possible alternative treatments for refractory cases.

De novo *absence status epilepticus of late onset*
This condition may develop in adult (usually elderly) patients, sometimes without a history of epilepsy. It presents as acute confusion and usually follows drug (especially benzodiazepine) withdrawal. It is important to consider this rare but treatable syndrome in the differential diagnosis of confusion in the elderly.

Electrical status epilepticus during slow wave sleep
This condition is difficult to diagnose unless sleep EEGs are recorded. It is most likely to complicate severe childhood epilepsies, especially those with cognitive symptomatology. Treatment is not considered to be an emergency. It is, however, thought that the cognitive difficulties are worsened through an alteration of sleep patterns. Valproate, lamotrigine, oral benzodiazepines and sometimes a course of steroids have been reported to be helpful.

Eclampsia

Eclampsia is unique to pregnancy. It occurs particularly in poorly nourished, young primigravidas or elderly multigravidas. It follows pre-eclampsia (hypertension and proteinuria) and manifests as headache, epileptic seizures and visual hallucinations (*eclampsia* Greek 'to shine forth').

Marked hypertension exceeds the limit of cerebral perfusion autoregulation, leading to cerebral oedema and cortical petechial haemorrhages. MR brain scanning shows marked cortical and white matter (especially occipital) high-signal abnormalities.

Management is to terminate the pregnancy and treat the woman urgently with antihypertensives, anticonvulsants and steroids. Magnesium sulphate, used since 1902, is superior to phenytoin or diazepam in the management of eclamptic seizures (Nielson, 1995). The prognosis with rapid intervention is excellent.

Cognitive and psychiatric aspects

Introduction

The major aspects of cognitive and psychiatric problems affecting people with epilepsy, or apparent epilepsy, are as follows:

- psychogenic non-epileptic attack disorder;
- learning disability;
- psychiatric difficulties in adults and children with epilepsy;
- behavioural effects of anti-epileptic medication.

Psychogenic attacks

Seizures, in the broadest sense, can occur in conditions other than epilepsy. Psychogenic non-epileptic seizures present a major diagnostic problem for doctors dealing with epilepsy. Up to 20 per cent of patients with a diagnostic label of epilepsy do not have epilepsy (Gates *et al.*, 1991), a large proportion of these having a psychological cause for their apparent blackouts. More worryingly, up to 50 per cent of patients in hospital with a diagnosis of status epilepticus do not have epilepsy (Howell *et al.*, 1989).

These figures emphasize the importance of a positive diagnosis of epilepsy at the outset, upon which management decisions can be based. It is almost always better to make no diagnosis than to reach an erroneous diagnosis of epilepsy.

TYPES OF PSYCHOGENIC ATTACK

Just as it is inappropriate to consider epilepsy as a single condition, so there are several types of psychogenic attack. The descriptive terms for non-epileptic seizures vary considerably. Hysteria, originally referring to womb movement as the cause of the symptoms, is clearly inappropriate and pejorative. 'Pseudoseizures', impling the attacks are 'not real', is judgemental and provokes communication difficulties in explaining attacks to patients.

The terms 'non-epileptic seizures' to describe the attacks, and 'non-epileptic attack disorder' (NEAD) to describe the patient's disorder are more acceptable and permit a better dialogue with the patient. 'Non-epileptic attack disorder' should actually include any condition characterized by attacks that are not primarily epileptic, such as syncope and cataplexy; in general, however, the term is used synonymously with psychogenic NEAD, and more particularly with dissociative NEAD ('pseudoseizures').

The two main groups of psychogenic NEAD are:

1. **panic disorder**, in which anxiety and hyperventilation lead to symptoms that can resemble seizures;
2. **dissociative disorder**, formerly known as 'pseudoseizures', in which a dissociation (conversion) disorder leads to behavioural disturbances that resemble epileptic seizures.

The two conditions overlap, and both lie along a single spectrum.

Panic disorder

Anxiety is an almost invariable accompaniment of a diagnosis of epilepsy and is sometimes responsible for the majority of a patient's symptoms. Considerable diagnostic confusion may result from three factors.

Panic symptoms resemble seizures

A very careful history is required to distinguish panic symptoms from complex partial seizures. Epileptic seizures are generally of sudden onset and stereotyped, with an aura followed by altered consciousness, automatism and then drowsiness and confusion. Panic symptoms are more gradual in onset and are accompanied by increasing anxiety. Important similarities are as follows:

- a gradual build-up of anxiety with 'frightened' epigastric sensations, tight feelings in the throat and palpitation;
- hyperventilation symptoms including breathlessness, chest tightness, sighing, tingling in the limbs and face (often unilateral), blurred vision and feeling distant and light headed;
- loss of consciousness (syncope with rapid recovery) may follow severe hyperventilation.

Panic symptoms exacerbate epilepsy

Hyperventilation lowers the threshold for epileptic seizures. This is well recognized in childhood absence epilepsy, in which seizures may be provoked by deliberate overbreathing in the clinic. Hyperventilation is used to bring out covert epileptiform activity on an EEG in any patient with suspected epilepsy. Recurrent hyperventilation in a patient with epilepsy may therefore increase the seizure frequency. A worsening of seizures at times of stress is still quite consistent with the diagnosis of epilepsy.

The **disrupted sleep pattern** accompanying anxiety may worsen epilepsy. A loss of sleep is well known to worsen epilepsy, especially the idiopathic forms. Patients with juvenile myoclonic epilepsy, for example, are advised to observe a regular sleep pattern for optimal seizure control. Sleep-deprived EEG recording is a useful technique to bring out covert abnormalities.

Panic disorder may be caused by epilepsy

The thought of having a seizure, often with little warning, in company and with the risk of injury and social stigma may provoke considerable and understandable anxiety. The resulting panic symptoms may resemble seizures. This can start a vicious circle of apparently increasing seizure frequency, the medical response often being to increase the anti-epileptic medication.

Case report

A 9-year-old boy gave a 2-year history of nocturnal left-sided face and arm jerking, diagnosed as benign childhood epilepsy with centrotemporal spikes. Having been well controlled on medication, he started to experience frequent daytime attacks, manifesting as tingling in the left hand and face with light-headedness, tremor and feeling distant from his surroundings. Some attacks were accompanied by breathlessness and choking sensations. Both the child and his parents became increasingly anxious about his apparently worsening epilepsy, resistant to increases in medication. Following a recognition of panic disorder and an explanation of the symptoms, the attacks resolved.

How to manage panic disorder

The aims of treatment are to:

- reduce the symptoms of the panic attacks;
- reduce the patient's anxiety;
- avoid provoking or 'threatening' situations.

General measures

A careful explanation of the nature of the anxiety attacks and the mechanism of symptom production is paramount. Written material on the mechanism and control of hyperventilation is often helpful.

Medication

Medication (e.g. beta blockers) may be used in the short term to control the symptoms of panic. Benzodiazepines, although not subjected to clinical trials for panic disorder, appear to help the symptoms and may assist in seizure control, although dependence upon medication may become a problem. Antidepressant medications, for example selective serotonin reuptake inhibitors such as paroxetine, may be useful, especially if combined with the psychological treatments outlined below (de Beurs *et al.*, 1995; DTB, 1997). Tricyclic antidepressants are, however, best avoided in patients with epilepsy, as they may lower the threshold for seizures.

Psychological treatments

Behavioural therapy focuses upon overcoming the avoidance behaviour rather than the panic itself. The patient is gradually introduced to a hierarchy of the feared situations with advice on measures to help to control the anxiety symptoms.

Cognitive behavioural therapy focuses upon the patient's tendency to misinterpret bodily sensations, for example palpitations or tingling, as indicating impending catastrophe. This tendency may have set up a vicious circle by increasing anxiety, provoking more anxiety symptoms and leading to a panic attack. Helping the patient to recognize and change this process can prevent the development of symptoms. Combined with breathing control or relaxation techniques (including aromatherapy), the symptoms may be overcome.

Outcome

Panic disorder, once recognized, can usually be treated successfully.

Dissociative non-epileptic attack disorder ('pseudoseizures')

Non-epileptic attacks mimicking tonic-clonic seizures (convulsive psychogenic non-epileptic seizures) present a major diagnostic difficulty as well as having significant resource implications and potential morbidity if the diagnosis is missed. Dissociative NEAD is relatively common and may account for up to 50 per cent of acute hospital admissions for supposed status epilepticus.

How to recognize dissociative NEAD ('pseudoseizures')

Attack characteristics

As with any seizure or blackout, the history is crucial to the diagnosis. Psychogenic non-epileptic seizures occur frequently despite medication and are typically provoked by stressful events. This gives the clinician a good opportunity to witness an attack. The seizures appear at first sight to

	Dissociative non-epileptic seizures ('pseudoseizures')	Epileptic seizures
Situational, e.g. anger, frustration	Common	Rare
May be induced by suggestion	Common	Less common
Onset	Often gradual	Usually sudden
Duration	Often prolonged	Seconds or minutes
Retained consciousness	Common	Rare
Pelvic thrusting and back arching (Fig. 7.1)	Common	Rare
Erratic movement, especially of the arms	Common	Rare
Fighting, needs to be held down, may injure others	Common	Rare
Eyes closed	Common	Less common
Resisting eye opening and eye contact	Common	Rare
Occur only in company	Common	Rare
Tongue biting and injury	Rare (occasional lip biting)	Common
Incontinence	Common in experienced patients	Common
Post-ictal confusion or drowsiness	Rare	Common

be very similar to epileptic seizures, but several features help to distinguish them (Table 7.1).

Table 7.1
Characteristics of dissociative non-epileptic seizures ('pseudoseizures') compared with epileptic seizures

Patient characteristics

Characteristics favouring a diagnosis of dissociative NEAD are:

- female (8:1 F:M);
- a history of resistant epilepsy beginning after the age of 10 years;
- previous episodes of status epilepticus;
- previous multiple hospital admissions, for example with self-harm, 'nervous asthma', irritable bowel or non-cardiac chest pain;
- a previous history of abnormal illness behaviour;
- a history of childhood physical and/or sexual abuse (Alper *et al.*, 1993).

How to confirm the diagnosis

Investigations are expected to be normal in dissociative NEAD.

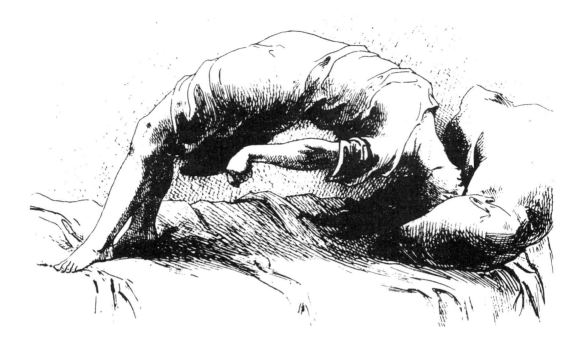

Figure 7.1
Dissociative non-epileptic attack disorder, showing the characteristic back arching ('*arc de cercle*') (drawing by Paul Richer, reproduced with permission).

Interictal EEG

The interictal EEG is likely to be normal. The diagnosis is essentially clinical, and it is important that undue emphasis is not be placed upon minor EEG changes. Patients with dissociative NEAD have often had an EEG purporting to show abnormalities that are erroneously interpreted in support of a diagnosis of epilepsy.

The EEG following a event is helpful in that the abnormal slowing expected after an epileptic seizure is absent immediately following a non-epileptic seizure.

Video EEG monitoring

Video EEG monitoring is particularly useful in dissociative NEAD, for several reasons:

- The attacks themselves can be observed and studied.
- The EEG accompanying the episodes can be seen to be normal (movement artefact only).
- The recording can be played back to the patient as part of the 'confrontation process', allowing a discussion of the thoughts and feelings experienced during the episode.

Prolactin

The blood prolactin level before and 20 minutes after the *onset* of an attack may add further information since an elevation of 10-fold would be expected following an epileptic convulsion and of 3–4-fold following a complex partial seizure. No significant rise follows a non-epileptic seizure.

Psychogenic status epilepticus (status pseudoepilepticus)

It is relatively common for patients with dissociative NEAD ('pseudo-seizures') to present to the emergency department with recurrent uncontrolled attacks.

In **psychogenic status epilepticus**, there is a discordance between the apparent severity of the epilepsy and the absence of significant brain disease. Major convulsions proving difficult to control in the face of no significant underlying brain disease must raise the suspicion of dissociative NEAD.

True status epilepticus usually occurs as a one-off event associated with significant acute brain dysfunction (e.g. encephalitis) or structural lesions (e.g. a frontal lobe tumour). Tonic-clonic seizures are usually quickly controlled using modern anti-epileptic medication.

True recurrent status epilepticus and severe epilepsy would be expected to be associated with at least one of the following:

- an onset before the age of 10 years;
- significant learning disability;
- significant neurological handicap;
- brain scan abnormality;
- significant EEG abnormality.

A patient apparently in status epilepticus with none of these characteristics must come under suspicion of having psychogenic status epilepticus.

How to manage dissociative NEAD

The usual first principle of clinical management is to obtain certainty of diagnosis. In dissociative NEAD, this involves proving a negative. It is rarely possible to be absolutely certain that a patient does not have epilepsy or that some of the attacks are epileptic and some are not. It is appropriate and helpful to discuss this element of diagnostic doubt with the patient.

The 'confrontation process'

Direct confrontation, or being dismissive or accusatory about the nature of the attacks, is rarely successful. A positive approach to the discussion of the diagnosis is helpful, with the patient being allowed to save face. The physician must explain several points to the patient:

- The clinical and investigation findings have suggested that the diagnosis is not epilepsy.
- This is good news as it implies that the condition is potentially curable.
- The attacks are real and disabling but probably have an emotional rather than an epileptic basis.
- The brain and nervous system produce many responses automatically and subconsciously, for example in breathing and heart rate; the seizures appear also to be a subconscious response of which the patient may be unaware.
- The attacks are as serious and disrupting as epilepsy but need a different form of treatment.
- Medications have not helped and may even be harmful; a fresh approach is needed.
- The EEG shows that the patient is awake during the attack – what thoughts are occurring during the episode?

Follow-up

Regular follow-up in the epilepsy clinic environment should be continued, with an opportunity to talk about problems and to voice fears and memories. The issue of childhood physical or sexual abuse may need to be addressed. One should not hurry to stop medication altogether since this can lead to feelings of rejection and loss of face.

Psychological management

As in panic disorder, a psychological approach including relaxation techniques, breathing control, hypnosis, aromatherapy or cognitive therapy may be beneficial.

Outcome

Dissociative NEAD is less easy to treat than panic disorder and is usually considered to have a poor prognosis. Handled sympathetically, however, and with long-term follow-up, there is the potential for a good outcome. Most cases can be treated, but it takes time. Cases diagnosed but quickly discharged do badly, either presenting the same problem to other doctors or hospitals, or developing new abnormal illness behaviours.

Morbidity

Many doctors regard dissociative NEAD as a time-consuming but nonetheless fairly harmless condition. There is, in fact, a significant morbidity attached to the condition, particularly when it mimics status epilepticus. Unnecessary and potentially harmful medications, and intervention of doctors in psychogenic status epilepticus, may lead to inappropriate intensive care, central lines, infection risk, assisted ventilation and even respiratory arrest. Psychogenic status epilepticus in pregnancy presents a particular hazard to the unborn child in terms of potentially teratogenic medications and the risk of premature intervention and delivery owing to resistant seizures.

Case report

A 24-year-old woman presented with an 18-month history of recurrent seizures resistant to anti-epileptic medication, requiring three admissions to intensive care in 'status' during the preceding year. She had also frequently been admitted for asthma. When 28 weeks into her third pregnancy, she developed recurrent seizures diagnosed as status epilepticus. Emergency caesarean section was advised, and the baby died after 2 hours. During a subsequent pregnancy, dissociative NEAD was diagnosed, and she acknowledged that the attacks were non-epileptic. Appropriate psychological treatment was instituted, the medication was discontinued and the attacks were brought under control, with the successful delivery of a healthy child (Smith *et al.*, 1999).

Is there epilepsy as well?

This is a very important question to ask when managing any patient with non-epileptic seizures. The traditional view is that some patients with epilepsy learn attention-seeking devices, which leads to a mixture of epileptic and non-epileptic seizures. However, this probably applies to only a minority of patients with NEAD.

Panic disorder is frequently the result of epilepsy (*see* above) so is frequently seen in patients with an established diagnosis of epilepsy. Equally importantly, as outlined above, it may be the sole cause of the patient's symptoms, with major implications for management.

Dissociative NEAD, particularly the convulsive form presenting as recurrent and resistant status pseudoepilepticus, commonly occurs in patients who have only ever had a behavioural disorder and who have never had epilepsy. This runs contrary to traditional teaching and accounts for much misdiagnosis and unnecessary treatment.

Do patients have non-epileptic seizures deliberately?

- **Panic disorder.** In patients with panic disorder, the panic symptoms can resemble complex partial seizures to both the patient and the physician; they are subconsciously generated and very alarming to the patient.
- **Dissociative NEAD.** At the other end of the spectrum, dissociative NEAD can be considered as an extreme form of body language expressing deep inner turmoil that the patient is otherwise unable to express.

The attacks are a manifestation of distress and are themselves distressing; it is difficult to believe that they are consciously generated. Deliberate malingering and Munchausen syndrome do present as NEAD but are rare.

Epilepsy misdiagnosed as NEAD

Patients with epilepsy are sometimes misdiagnosed as having NEAD, especially in the following situations:

- **Medial temporal lobe seizures** typically begin with epigastric 'butterflies' and may be accompanied by other non-specific, panic-like symptoms suggesting panic disorder.
- **Frontal lobe seizures** arising in the supplementary motor area may cause recurrent shaking and tonic episodes with retained consciousness and even a normal EEG during attacks, suggesting dissociative NEAD.
- **Parietal lobe seizures** presenting as episodic lateralized sensations or pain without any motor component may be dismissed as NEAD.
- **Occipital lobe seizures** may give seemingly bizarre symptoms such as ictal blindness or visual hallucinations, which are easily labelled as functional.
- **Stress and epilepsy.** A seizure tendency may worsen at times of stress (anxiety, with sleep loss or premenstrually). Epilepsy itself is stressful so may worsen an anxiety tendency. Thus, identifying significant stress does not necessarily suggest that the diagnosis is not epilepsy.

Learning disability

Learning disability may be either global or specific. **Specific learning disability** is characterized by defined areas of difficulty leading to, for example, dyslexia or dyscalculia. **Global learning disability** is defined as a full-scale intelligence quotient (IQ) of less than 2 standard deviations below the mean; it thus represents the extreme of a continuum.

One-third of the people who have learning disabilities also have epilepsy, and at least one-quarter of those with epilepsy have additional cognitive problems. On the whole, those who have learning disabilities tend to have more severe epilepsy; the epilepsy responds less well to medication, and consequently their difficulties are compounded. Many have additional physical difficulties such as cerebral palsy.

Learning disability in epilepsy can be considered from three main aspects:

- the effects of underlying brain disorders responsible for both the epilepsy and the learning difficulties;

- the effects of the seizures themselves;
- the effects of medication.

EFFECTS OF UNDERLYING BRAIN DISORDERS ON LEARNING ABILITIES

Disorders of the brain associated with both epilepsy and cognitive problems may largely be classified as congenital or acquired. However, some metabolic disorders, such as those associated with peroxisomal dysfunction (e.g. Zellweger syndrome), straddle the sharp division between truly prenatal and postnatal aetiologies.

Predominantly congenital disorders causing learning disability and epilepsy

There are three groups of congenital disorders in which learning difficulties and epilepsy co-exist.

Neuronal migration disorders

Abnormalities of neuronal migration (*see* Chapter 3), when severe and generalized, such as in lissencephaly, are inevitably associated with profound learning disability and epilepsy. The spectrum of severity of migrational disorders is wide, with a comparable diversity in the severity of learning difficulties. Epilepsy can remain a significant problem even if only small zones of heterotopic neurones are visible. The degree of migrational abnormality is related more directly to the learning disability than to the severity of the epilepsy. Malformations of cortical development involving aberrations of the stages of cortical development (i.e. those other than migrational disorders) are more likely to lead to uncomplicated global cognitive difficulties.

Intracerebral cysts

Intracerebral cysts follow prenatal intracerebral vascular occlusion with subsequent infarction and later the formation of a cyst, the wall of which often contains epileptogenic material. Affected infants are likely to have lateralized motor disabilities and lateralized seizures, with specific learning difficulties, although the latter can be global.

Chromosomal abnormalities

Epilepsy and learning disability may co-exist in people who have chromosomal abnormalities, recognizable on cytogenetic testing and *in situ* hybridization.

Several epilepsies for which genes have been identified have been considered in Chapter 5. Further information on the clinical features of the following conditions can be found in Smith and Jones (1996).

Sex chromosome abnormalities   Additional sex chromosomes have been identified in individuals with both learning difficulties and epilepsy. Those with XXY, XYY and XXX chromosomes have a greater than usual risk of epilepsy. Although learning and behavioural difficulties are the usual expressions of fragile X syndrome, a trinucleotide p(CCG)n repeat within the *FMR-1* gene at Xq 27.3 also gives an increased propensity to epilepsy; this occurs in about 25 per cent of cases.

Angelman and Prader–Willi syndromes   In both syndromes, there is typically a deletion in one chromosome at 15q11–13. If the deletion is in the paternally derived chromosome 15, Prader–Willi syndrome results, with learning disability but rarely epilepsy. If the deletion is in the maternally derived chromosome 15, Angelman syndrome, with severe learning difficulties, occurs and additional epilepsy is usual. The seizures are likely to be atypical absence, atonic and myoclonic in type and are often difficult to treat. Either Prader–Willi or Angelman syndrome may also occur if there is uniparental disomy for chromosome 15, i.e. if two chromosomes 15 are inherited from either the mother or father, rather than one from each parent. In these circumstances, Angelman syndrome presents if the two chromosomes 15 are paternal and Prader–Willi syndrome if they are of maternal origin.

Other chromosomal deletions and rearrangements   Deletions have been recognized in association with the Miller–Dieker, Smith–Magenis, Wolf–Hirschhorn and Pallister–Killian syndromes. Other chromosomal deletions, mutations or duplications will, no doubt, be associated with further syndromes of learning difficulty with epilepsy in the future. The gene for Rett syndrome (*see* Chapter 4), in which epilepsy occurs in 75 per cent of cases, has now been identified at Xq28.

Trisomies   Epilepsy is up to 10 times more common in Down's syndrome, trisomy 21, than expected; in childhood, there is an increased risk of infantile spasms. Trisomy 12p and trisomy 13 (Patall's syndrome) are also associated with epilepsy. In those with a ring chromosome 14, seizures start in early infancy.

Acquired or later-onset disorders of learning disability and epilepsy

Acquired or later-onset conditions in which learning disability and epilepsy co-exist are divisible into two main groups:

- metabolic/biochemical disturbances and conditions associated with dementia;
- direct brain injuries leading to localized or more generalized structural abnormalities.

Metabolic/biochemical disturbances

Inborn errors of metabolism associated with epilepsy are listed in Table 5.3 (p. 108). Such conditions are almost invariably associated with poor cognitive development or a loss of intellectual skills. However, neonatal hypoglycaemia, hypocalcaemia and hypomagnesaemia, fatty acid oxidation defects, mitochondrial disorders and porphyria do not necessarily have implications for learning.

Hypoglycaemia that is severe and recurring, associated with insulin treatment for diabetes mellitus, can be followed by epilepsy and learning difficulties.

Asphyxial brain damage in the neonatal period, and at later times, when it may be associated with drowning, suffocation, strangulation, etc., is likely to cause both learning disabilities and epilepsy.

Secondary metabolic changes may occur. Some of the damage done by direct head injuries, such as those consequent on road traffic accidents, is probably asphyxial in nature, being secondary to shock and poor generalized cerebral perfusion.

Dementing conditions of the later years are associated with an increased risk of epilepsy. Seizures occur in 10 per cent of patients with Alzheimer's disease.

Direct brain injuries

- **Trauma.** Epilepsy secondary to traumatic head injury has been considered in detail in Chapter 3. Learning disability may clearly also be acquired.
- **Infection.** Encephalitis, and to a lesser extent meningitis, can be followed by both epilepsy and cognitive problems.

EFFECTS OF THE SEIZURES THEMSELVES ON LEARNING ABILITIES

Seizures may affect cognitive abilities by two mechanisms:

- causing localized or generalized toxicity to neurones;
- interfering with the processing of information.

Toxic effects

These may be primary or secondary. Primary effects involve the production of excitotoxic amino acids and interference with ion channel function.

Secondary effects are those of a more general nature related to asphyxia and are thus more likely to be relevant to generalized tonic-clonic status epilepticus.

The risks of both primary and secondary effects increase directly with the duration of seizures. Although the brains of neonates are considered to be more resistant to seizure damage than those of older children, there is some evidence that global cognitive disabilities are most likely to occur if convulsive status epilepticus presents in the first year of life.

Interference with the processing of information

Transient cognitive impairment

Simultaneous video and EEG recordings have made it possible to identify very brief lapses in attention, which occur during isolated epileptic spike discharges. Such lapses can be most readily demonstrated when subjects are performing tasks that either require little concentration or they find difficult. A degree of concentration, without accompanying anxiety about the task, tends to reduce the frequency of isolated spike discharges.

Epilepsies with cognitive symptomatology

These have been considered in Chapter 3. Non-convulsive seizure disorders should be considered if there are fluctuating cognitive abilities, frequent mood changes, uneven memory skills or a marked variation in the ability to relate to the environment. The most common situation is interference with the receipt of information during childhood absence attacks. This epilepsy is, however, much more readily recognized than Landau–Kleffner and related syndromes, in which periods of abstraction may last for hours or even days. In childhood, electrical status epilepticus during slow wave sleep may produce a state comparable to dementia. Children with benign partial epilepsies may have specific learning problems such as dyslexia.

THE EFFECTS OF ANTI-EPILEPTIC DRUGS ON LEARNING ABILITIES

Anti-epileptic drugs might cause or contribute to learning disabilities. Non-medical members of the public, particularly teachers, often fuel such concerns, but they are in most cases ill founded.

- **Phenobarbitone.** In young children, there is some evidence that treatment with phenobarbitone may lead to a poor ability on tests of comprehension (Camfield *et al.*, 1980), but if given in doses that avoid sedation, there is little to suggest cognitive impairment.

- **Phenytoin** has been studied in both adults and children, with somewhat equivocal results. On the whole, the more sophisticated the study, the less convincing was the adverse effect on cognition.
- **Carbamazepine** seems to have no definite influence on learning abilities.
- **Valproate.** The dose of valproate could be important in determining whether or not cognitive side effects occur. Concentration, memory and motility have been reported to be less good at high than at low dosage (Aman *et al.*, 1987).
- **Vigabatrin** does not harm cognitive functions in adults (Gilham *et al.*, 1993) or children (Kalviainen *et al.*, 1991).
- **Oxcarbazepine** is not associated with significant cognitive changes.
- **Lamotrigine** does not adversely affect cognition in therapeutic doses and can even increase alertness as a result of a reduction in seizure discharges.

The behavioural effects of anti-epileptic drugs, commonly of more concern and definitely more frequent, are considered below.

Psychiatric difficulties with epilepsy

Epilepsy is closely linked to psychiatric disease, with many important overlaps existing that significantly influence the clinical assessment and management. The psychiatric problems associated with epilepsy can be considered as either 'ictal', arising as a direct consequence of a seizure, or 'interictal', arising in loose association with the epilepsy tendency.

ICTAL PSYCHIATRIC DISORDERS

The 'ictal' period, defined clinically rather than on the EEG, includes the duration of pre-ictal and post-ictal phenomena. During complex partial seizures, psychiatric phenomena such as hallucinations, illusions, perceptual disturbance and cognitive and affective disorders can occur.

INTERICTAL PSYCHIATRIC DISORDERS

The full spectrum of psychiatric disorders is seen in the epilepsy patient population, ranging from depression, anxiety, personality disorder and hysterical phenomena, to cognitive impairment and schizophreniform illness. Most reports have concerned populations in psychiatric institutions, thus over-representing the more serious psychotic disorders. A community survey (Edeh and Toone, 1987), however, showed that, although psychiatric disorders are twice as common in the epilepsy population compared with the

Case report

A 20-year-old woman with a history of complex partial seizures was admitted with confusion 2 days after a secondary generalized seizure. Since the convulsion, she had become increasingly paranoid, fearing that her parents were trying to harm her and her 2-year-old child; she resisted examination by the doctor and threatened self-discharge. She showed expressive dysphasia and mild right-sided facial weakness but no other lateralizing neurological signs. Her EEG showed a generalized excess of slow waveforms, particularly left sided, without specific 'epileptic' activity; a magnetic resonance brain scan was normal. Her usual anti-epileptic medication was continued, and her condition improved over 3 days; at a clinic follow-up after 2 weeks, she had made a full recovery, with excellent insight into her condition. A diagnosis of postictal paranoid psychosis was made.

general population, anxiety and depression predominate, and psychotic problems are rare.

Stress and epilepsy

People with epilepsy understandably experience an increased amount of stress. Not only are they naturally fearful of having a seizure with little or no warning, causing embarrassment and injury, but also their condition frequently provokes fear and hostility among friends, colleagues, employers and the general public. Low self-esteem and social isolation are common consequences of epilepsy. In addition, their medication may induce sedative or cosmetic side effects (including weight gain), adding to their anxiety.

Stress is a significant factor in exacerbating epilepsy and may itself give rise to episodes that both the patient and physician can confuse with seizures (*see* above).

Chronic psychoses of epilepsy

Although rare, the chronic psychoses of epilepsy are of considerable interest and have led to speculation that discharges similar to epileptic discharges in the limbic system might account for some psychotic disease:

- A **schizophreniform illness** is the classical manifestation of epilepsy psychosis, usually deriving from dominant hemisphere medial temporal lesions.
- The **Geschwind syndrome** (usually a non-dominant hemisphere problem) comprises hypergraphia, hyper-religiosity and hyposexuality. Vincent van Gogh is considered by some to have exhibited this condition (Trimble,

1991), his hypergraphia manifesting as an enormous output of artistic as well as written material.

Mechanisms of epilepsy-related psychiatric disorder

There are several possible mechanisms by which psychiatric disorders might arise in patients with epilepsy.

Even in apparently seizure-free patients, it may be that **seizures** themselves are causing the psychosis. Interictal EEG changes or 'subclinical' seizures potentially detectable on depth EEG electrode recordings may be inducing limbic dysfunction. Patients with localization-related epilepsy are at greater risk of such problems than those with generalized epilepsies.

Seizures themselves can presumably cause psychosis through neurochemical changes. The benefit of electroconvulsive therapy to certain psychotic disorders is therefore ironic, leaving the mechanism open to question.

Forced normalization may occur. New psychiatric symptoms sometimes develop in patients with previously poor seizure control and coincide with seizure control on medication.

Severe brain damage is commonly associated with epilepsy and is likely to be the main reason why patients with severe epilepsy, as well as patients with other organic brain disorders, develop psychotic symptoms.

Genetic factors strongly influence the development of epilepsy. There is also a considerable overlap between genetically determined epilepsy and learning disability. Many of the single gene epilepsy disorders (*see* Chapter 5) are associated with significant neurodevelopmental problems and handicap.

Psychosocial factors are the main mechanism by which neurotic disorders arise in patients with epilepsy. Social stresses, problems with the attitude of family and peer groups, disturbed relationships and social stigma, together with difficulties with employment and driving, all contribute.

PSYCHIATRIC ASPECTS IN CHILDREN

Seizures in childhood, as in adults, can present with psychiatric or behavioural manifestations, either subjective or objective:

- **Subjective** manifestations are related to abnormal sensations, hallucinations, and illusions.
- **Objective** manifestations include identifiable behavioural changes.

The differentiation between primary behavioural and primary seizure manifestations can be very difficult, particularly if the patient is very young or learning disabled. Many children with epilepsy, particularly those with additional cognitive problems, have obvious difficulty in learning to behave in socially acceptable ways.

SPECIFIC PSYCHIATRIC DISORDERS IN CHILDREN

A few childhood psychiatric disorders merit particular consideration in the context of epilepsy (Taylor, 1996).

Psychoses

- **Autism** or autistic spectrum disorders may follow infantile spasms or Lennox–Gastaut syndrome. In addition, epilepsy may present in later childhood or adolescence in those already considered to be autistic. It has been suggested that, in these cases, both epilepsy and autism represent a neurodevelopmental abnormality within the limbic system.
- **Asperger's syndrome** may be associated with seizures. In some cases, neuronal migration defects can be found on neuro-imaging.
- **Schizophrenia** is rare in childhood but may present in later life, particularly following epilepsy of temporal lobe origin.

Affective disorders

These are rare in prepubertal children, but 'depression' may be related in part to an inadequate control of seizures.

Suicide

Attempts at suicide are increased in adolescents with epilepsy, when compared with their seizure-free peers.

Hyperkinesis

Epilepsy is over-represented in children with the attention deficit hyperactivity disorder. Females with this condition are more likely to have epilepsy, even though more males have the condition.

Conduct disorder

Children with epilepsy are not always well liked by other children, being perceived as irritable and resentful when corrected, and as having tics, mannerisms and a tendency to squirm and fidget. There have, however, been difficulties with assessing information provided from different sources, for example parents and school, since preconceived perceptions may flaw the validity of questionnaires.

Obsessions

Individuals with epilepsy may have extreme obsessions. Taylor (1996) reports elements of Tourette's syndrome, Asperger's syndrome and compulsive disorder in several patients with epilepsy.

Neuroses

Fears, worries, miseries, etc. are generally more common in children with epilepsy.

Non-epileptic attack disorder

In childhood, NEAD exists in two forms:

- **Dissociation.** Unconsciousness as a form of behaviour, a type of opting-out mechanism, is usually secondary to extreme distress. Young subjects of unwelcome sexual interest may express their problems in this way.
- **Meadow syndrome** (Munchausen syndrome by proxy). In this, there is an imposition of a physical diagnosis, such as epilepsy, either by direct means, for example suffocation, or by a fictitious presentation of the history.

Behavioural effects of anti-epileptic drugs

Following the introduction of some anti-epileptic drugs, behavioural disturbances are more consistently recognized than cognitive effects:

- **Phenobarbitone** is associated in at least 25 per cent of young children with overactive behaviour. Poor attention skills, irritability and disturbed sleep patterns co-exist. Drowsiness and lethargy occur at high doses.
- **Phenytoin.** Drowsiness and lethargy are dose related.
- **Carbamazepine.** Drowsiness may occur on introduction of the drug and at a high dosage. Some studies in children have suggested that behaviour can be improved.
- **Valproate.** Adverse behavioural effects including overactivity have been reported anecdotally but are not confirmed in formal studies. Increased appetite can lead to hyperphagia and consequent excessive weight gain.
- **Lamotrigine.** The effects on behaviour are usually positive. Adult patients often describe a feeling of improved well-being. In a paediatric study of lamotrigine in Lennox–Gastaut syndrome, a questionnaire suggested an improvement in quality of life additional to that noted for seizure control.
- **Gabapentin.** Somnolence may occur, but, on the whole, behavioural difficulties do not occur in adults on gabapentin. There are reports of overactivity in a few children.

- **Topiramate.** Drowsiness can be a problem but is least likely with a low starting dose and a slow escalation, as necessary. Severe withdrawal behaviour, with apparent loss of skills, has been seen in small children; this is reversible if topiramate is discontinued.
- **Vigabatrin** may precipitate psychosis. Up to 10 per cent of adults develop mood changes, with agitation, ill-temper, disturbed behaviour or depression. Following the introduction of vigabatrin, children may become extremely drowsy or extremely active. The drowsiness is likely to improve, but overactivity, aggressiveness and insomnia may persist until vigabatrin is withdrawn.
- **Tiagabine.** Tiredness has been reported in adults, but there is very little information on behavioural effects in children.
- **Oxcarbazepine.** No major adverse effects on behaviour have been recorded.
- **Benzodiazepines.** The main problems relate to drowsiness. Occasional patients react with extreme disinhibition, including unprovoked aggression.

Epilepsy in special client groups

8

Seizures in the neonate (0–4 weeks)

DIFFERENTIAL DIAGNOSIS: NON-EPILEPTIC EVENTS

Confusion with other paroxysmal events is common in the neonate. In particular, other attacks in which disturbances of breathing and cardiovascular stability occur are often misdiagnosed as being epileptic in nature:

- **Clonus or segmental clonus** (tremulousness or jitteriness) may mimic multifocal or fragmentary generalized clonic seizures.
- **Stereotyped movements**, for example bicycling or chewing movements, can be due to brainstem release phenomena.
- **Parasympathetic features** such as bradycardia, increased peristalsis, increased tracheal secretions and miosis (resulting from parasympathetic discharges) are more likely to occur than seizure activity in neonatal encephalopathy.
- **Myoclonic jerks** occur exclusively in sleep in benign sleep myoclonus.
- **Hyperekplexia**, causing excessive startles, stiffness and apnoea, may resemble epilepsy.
- **Tonic posturing in extension** is more likely to be caused by functional decerebration than seizures.

EPIDEMIOLOGY

The overall incidence of seizures in the neonate is difficult to define accurately. In the past, some movement patterns, now recognized as being due to other causes, were wrongly considered to be epileptic in nature. In electroencephalographically confirmed seizures in neonates, the incidence was given as 2 per 1000 in 40 845 live-born infants (Scher *et al.*, 1993). Some groups of neonates are particularly vulnerable to seizures, the incidence being:

- 23 per 1000 of those admitted to the neonatal intensive care unit;
- 39 per 1000 of intensive care neonates of less than 31 weeks' gestation;

- 10 out of 32 (31 per cent) of infants born outside the reporting centre and transferred in because of illness (Scher *et al.*, 1993).

SEIZURE TYPES AND EPILEPSIES

Some information on neonatal seizures and epilepsies has already been presented (*see* Chapter 3). Owing to brain immaturity, seizure types in infants can differ from those seen in older children and adults.

A number of phenomena are regularly seen in association with EEG changes:

- subtle changes: ocular movements, with tonic horizontal deviation of the eyes, with or without jerking of the eyes, or with sustained eye opening and ocular fixation; oro-bucco-lingual movements, including chewing; limb movements; autonomic phenomena; apnoeic spells;
- focal, or multifocal, clonic attacks;
- focal tonic seizures;
- generalized myoclonic seizures.

Generalized and tonic attacks, as well as focal or multifocal myoclonic seizures, may rarely be associated with EEG changes. The neonatal brain seems insufficiently mature to produce classical generalized tonic-clonic seizures.

Infants of less than 31 weeks' gestation tend to have seizures lasting less than 30 minutes, with relatively short interictal periods. In contrast, more mature infants can sustain seizures for longer; and the duration of the interictal periods also tends to be greater.

The epilepsy syndromes that can start in the neonatal period (*see* Chapter 3) are:

- benign familial neonatal convulsions
- early myoclonic encephalopathy
- early infantile epileptic encephalopathy
- non-familial forms of benign neonatal convulsions.

AETIOLOGY

In the neonate, seizures are likely to be symptomatic. It is very important to diagnose the underlying condition since its treatment can be crucial to the long-term outlook. Hypoxic–ischaemic encephalopathy, intracerebral haemorrhage, cerebral malformation, infection and metabolic disturbance are the most prominent factors.

Hypoxic–ischaemic encephalopathy

Seizures usually present within 24 hours of birth, and always within 3 days. Deep stupor or coma, periodic breathing, hypotonia and additional renal and cardiac complications are common. Hypoglycaemia, hypocalcaemia, hypoxaemia and acidosis contribute to a severe clinical picture.

Intracerebral haemorrhage

Severe intracerebral haemorrhage is associated with generalized tonic seizures, but additional subtle events may occur.

Cerebral malformations

Seizures secondary to cerebral malformations usually, but not always, present after the neonatal period.

Infections

These can be considered to be prenatal, intranatal or immediately postnatal in acquisition:

- **Prenatal infectious agents** causing seizures include cytomegalovirus, rubella, toxoplasmosis, human immunodeficiency virus, Coxsackie B, echovirus, varicella and syphilis.
- **Intrapartum acquired infections** are those of herpes simplex (which can cause very persistent partial seizures as part of an encephalitic illness), Coxsackie B, group B streptococci, *Escherichia coli* and other enterics, *Listeria monocytogenes* and other staphylococci and streptococci.

Metabolic disturbances

These can can be considered in two groups:

- **Temporary disturbances** such as hypoglycaemia, hypocalcaemia, hypomagnesaemia, hypernatraemia and hyponatraemia.
- **Inborn errors of metabolism** (considered in Chapter 5). Those requiring consideration in the neonatal period are aminoacidopathies, organic acidopathies, urea cycle disorders, pyridoxine dependency and glucose transporter deficiency.

Withdrawal from maternal drugs

Seizures may follow withdrawal from maternal barbiturates, alcohol, heroin, cocaine or methadone. Irritability and tremor are, however, more common than seizures.

Local anaesthetic intoxication

Seizures, bradycardia and hypoventilation can be precipitated by the inadvertent injection of local anaesthetic into the infant scalp while preparing for instrumental delivery.

GENETICS

- **Benign familial neonatal convulsions.** This syndrome shows autosomal dominant inheritance at two gene locations, mapping to 20q13 and 8q24, the gene symbols being *KCNQ2* and *KCNQ3* respectively; the effect is on voltage-gated potassium channels.
- **Inborn errors of metabolism.** Genetic factors are particularly important when the seizures are secondary to inborn errors of metabolism. Most are autosomal recessive, but there are some X-linked exceptions, such as ornithine carbamylase transferase deficiency.

PATHOLOGY

Developmental issues create specific considerations. In the latter periods of gestation, glutamate receptors take part in activity-dependent synaptic development. Conversely, an overproduction of glutamate, as occurs in seizures, can lead to neuronal death. High concentrations of brain glutamate result from hypoxic–ischaemic states.

There is animal evidence that the neonatal brain is more resistant to seizure damage than that of older children. There is, however, no doubt that energy metabolism is affected by seizures and that hypoxia increases the risk of permanent brain damage.

NEUROPHYSIOLOGICAL INVESTIGATIONS

Particular skills are required in the interpretation of the neonatal EEG. There are gestation-related changes so that specific patterns may be normal in the premature neonate but abnormal by full term:

- **24–27 weeks.** The background activity is discontinuous, with long, flat stretches interspersed by short bursts of activity, a picture similar to that of suppression-burst in an older person.
- **28–31 weeks.** The background remains discontinuous, but periods of activity are beginning to predominate, although differences between sleep and waking have not yet developed.
- **32–35 weeks.** The background activity becomes continuous when awake and in rapid eye movement (REM) sleep but remains discontinuous during non-REM sleep (*tracé alternant*). The different patterns during non-REM and REM sleep are indications not only of gestation, but also of cerebral well-being. This differentiation tends to be lost in neonatal encephalopathies, even if frank seizures do not occur.
- **36–41 weeks.** There is a good differentiation between sleep and waking with *tracé alternant* persisting during non-REM sleep. Moderate voltage 1–3 Hz activity predominates during waking.

In keeping with brain immaturity, spikes are rare in the very premature but may accompany seizures in the more mature. Rhythmic slow waves, persistent focal sharp waves, repeated stereotyped sharp waves and slow wave complexes, small-amplitude waves and/or fast activity are all considered to be EEG evidence of seizures. It is usual to record neonatal EEGs by ambulatory monitoring for at least 1–2 hours so that the waking, REM and non-REM sleep patterns may all be assessed.

IMAGING

For sick immature infants, the easiest option is ultrasound scanning. Germinal matrix haemorrhage, hydrocephalus and other major brain mal-formations, especially those involving midline structures, can be seen. The addition of colour Doppler flow imaging allows the cortical pattern to be visualized.

However, if brain parenchymal disorders, haemorrhage into the subdural or subarachnoid space, or posterior fossa abnormalities are suspected, either computed tomography (CT) or magnetic resonance imaging (MRI) is needed. MRI is preferred since it allows a better definition of the maturation of myelination, disorders of neuronal migration and vascular abnormalities than does CT scanning.

MANAGEMENT

Correctable causes

It is essential to consider remediable precipitating events such as hypogly-caemia. The correction of metabolic disorders is paramount.

If pyridoxine dependency is suspected, give 50–100 mg pyridoxine intra-venously. If this is the cause of the seizures, both EEG and clinical seizures will stop during the injection. Therapy is needed lifelong.

Anti-epileptic medications

Phenobarbitone or phenytoin is the usual treatment:

- **Phenobarbitone** has a prolonged half-life in infants.
- **Phenytoin** is not absorbed adequately if given orally or nasogastrically in close association with milk feeds.
- **Lorazepam** could be the benzodiazepine of choice in neonatal seizures (Deshmukh *et al.*, 1986).
- **Diazepam** has variable effects in neonates, and its half-life is much longer in neonates than in older patients. Many preparations contain sodium benzoate, which may increase the level of unconjugated bilirubin.

Table 8.1
Anti-epileptic drug dosages for neonatal seizures

Drug	Loading dose	Infusion rate	Maintenance dose
Phenobarbitone	20 mg/kg intravenously		3–4 mg/kg/day
Phenytoin	20 mg/kg intravenously	Slow delivery	5–10 mg/kg/day related to plasma level
Clonazepam		10 µg/kg/hour	
Lorazepam	0.05–0.1 mg/kg intravenously over 2–5 minutes		
Lidocaine		4–60 mg/kg/hour	

- **Clonazepam**, given as an infusion, can be effective in seizures resistant to phenobarbitone or phenytoin.
- **Paraldehyde** intravenously was previously used in resistant cases, but non-availability has removed this option.
- **Lidocaine** given intravenously is a further possibility (Hellström-Westas *et al.*, 1988).

Appropriate dosages for these medications are given in Table 8.1.

PROGNOSIS FOR FURTHER SEIZURES/EPILEPSY

The underlying aetiology dictates the prognosis. Neonates with severe haemorrhages or major cerebral malformations are unlikely to survive. Of the survivors, at least 50 per cent are likely to continue to have seizures. Factors leading to the greatest risk are as follows:

- coma;
- significant disturbances of the background EEG;
- the later development of cerebral palsy or mental retardation;
- spikes and sharp and slow wave activity on postnatal follow-up EEGs.

COGNITIVE IMPLICATIONS

At least 20 per cent of neonates who have had seizures later show cognitive and learning difficulties. The most important predictive factor seems to be the amount of structural brain abnormality present rather than effects of the seizures themselves. Congenital malformations and hypoxic–ischaemic encephalopathy are most likely to be associated with later learning disorders. Benign familial and non-familial convulsions or readily correctable biochemical and metabolic disorders suggest a good outlook for cognitive development.

SOCIAL FACTORS

The presence of seizures in a neonate, particularly if associated with other evidence of cerebral dysfunction, is clearly a cause for concern regarding the long-term neurological outlook. It is important that reassurance is given to the parents where this is appropriate, i.e. in benign familial and non-familial convulsions and where a readily correctable biochemical or metabolic disorder has been identified. It is equally essential to give a guarded, but factual, prognosis when risk factors for subsequent epilepsy, cerebral palsy and learning difficulties are present, and to keep such infants under review with appropriate support until later development can be adequately assessed.

Seizures in the infant (4 weeks to 2 years)

FEBRILE SEIZURES

Seizures precipitated by febrile illnesses occur in approximately 5 per cent of all children and in about 15 per cent of those who have a febrile illness in the vulnerable age range.

Definition

Febrile seizures are usually defined as seizures of cerebral origin that occur in association with infections not involving the intracranial structures. However, although it may be clear whether or not bacterial or viral meningitis is present, the exclusion of encephalitis, particularly when this is mild, is more difficult. It is therefore more useful to consider all seizures precipitated by feverish illnesses as febrile seizures and to take note, as a separate issue, of the aetiology of the fever. The height of the fever considered appropriate for use of the term 'febrile seizure' is 38 °C. Many children with such seizures have minor neurological disabilities. It is not appropriate to exclude seizures in such children from the definition of a febrile seizure.

Differential diagnosis

The differential diagnosis is the same as for other seizures/epilepsies in this age range.

Age of onset

Age of onset is an important factor. Although the range of vulnerability extends between 6 months and 3 years, and thus beyond infancy, most affected children will have their first febrile seizure in the second year of life. Complex febrile seizures are more likely to occur in the first year than later.

Predisposing causes

Infection

Ninety per cent of precipitating infections are viral. Clinically, most involve the upper respiratory tract. However, bacterial urinary tract and meningeal infections must not be overlooked. In approximately 3 per cent of children who present with a fever and a seizure, bacterial meningitis is the cause. Urinary tract infections and unexpected pneumococcal bacteraemia are each found in about another 3 per cent. Shigellosis accounts for a few cases. Only 1.4 per cent of all febrile seizures follow vaccination.

Genetic factors

Genetic factors have been recognized for many years. The gene, *SCN1B*, for the syndrome of generalized epilepsy with febrile seizures plus (*see* Chapter 3) is located at 19q13, the gene product having been identified as the sodium channel beta-1 subunit. This is an autosomal dominant condition.

Other locations and gene symbols are possibly 8q13–21 for *FEB 1*, 19q13.3 for *FEB 2*, 2q23–24 for *FEB 3*, and 5q14–15 for *FEB 4*. These four situations are involved in complex modes of inheritance, and the gene products have not been identified. For practical purposes, there is a higher risk of febrile seizures in the children of parents who have a history of febrile seizures or epilepsy.

Other predisposing factors

- **Prenatal:** during pregnancy, chronic maternal illness, smoking and a high alcohol intake, repeated early small vaginal bleeds and toxaemia.
- **Perinatal:** delivery by other than the vertex and a relative reduction in birth weight for gestation.
- **Postnatal:** prior to the initial febrile seizure, a significant increase in infective illnesses has been shown. At least 20–25 per cent of affected children have a minor deviation from a totally normal neurodevelopmental history.

Adverse prenatal and perinatal events increase the risk that any seizure occurring will be complex. Prior neurological disturbance, even if mild, also predisposes to complex febrile seizures, as well as to febrile status epilepticus.

Seizure characteristics

'Simple' febrile seizures are defined as generalized and brief, i.e. of less than 15 minutes' duration.

'Complex' febrile seizures last 15 minutes or more and/or are partial or lateralized at some time in their evolution, and/or are repeated within the same illness.

The characterization of the first seizure is the most important guide to the long-term prognosis.

- **Lateralized seizures** suggest prior neurological dysfunction.
- **Prolonged seizures.** In the acute postictal phase, a prolonged disturbance of consciousness should suggest an underlying intracranial infection.
- **Asymmetrical motor function** indicates that there were prior neurological problems and/or that the seizure had lateralizing features.
- **Hemiparesis.** An acute, usually transient, hemiparesis (Todd's paresis) following a prolonged, lateralized febrile seizure is of particular significance for the later development of complex partial seizures.

Investigation

Investigation at presentation is chiefly aimed at identifying the underlying infection. EEGs do not help with the prognosis, nor do they help in managing the acute illness. Thus, febrile seizures are the only situation in which an EEG would not be arranged after a seizure.

Management

The **acute therapy** is the same as for any other seizure disorder, intravenous lorazepam or rectal diazepam being the initial choice and progression to other measures occurring as indicated in Chapter 6. The parents of those in whom there is an increased risk of recurrence should be given instruction in antipyretic measures and supplied with rectal preparations of diazepam to be given should the child have a further seizure that does not terminate spontaneously within 2–3 minutes.

Continuous prophylactic therapy is rarely given after a first or second febrile seizure, even when the risk of recurrence is high, but if more than three or four seizures have occurred and the child is still well within the vulnerable age range, regular anti-epileptic drug therapy should be considered, valproate being the usual choice.

Prognosis

Seizure recurrence

A **recurrence of febrile seizures** occurs in approximately 30–40 per cent of children who have a single such seizure. The risk is related to defined factors, each of which, when summated, increases the likelihood:

- low social class
- young age, particularly less than 12 months
- seizure disorders in first-degree relatives
- continuing neurological disorders
- a complex initial febrile seizure.

The recurrence risk is about 15 per cent when none of these factors is present and rises by approximately 15 per cent for each item, so that children with all of the adverse features almost invariably have further febrile seizures.

Non-febrile seizures and epilepsy may develop. Children who have had a febrile seizure have a significant risk of subsequent non-febrile seizures and epilepsy. The risk of unprovoked seizures is 7 per cent by the age of 25 years. In 85 per cent of cases, unprovoked seizures will start within 4 years, but much longer intervals have been reported. Progression to a defined epilepsy syndrome is rare but has been noted for virtually all syndromes with an onset after the first year. On the whole, localization-related epilepsies follow lateralized seizures. Brief generalized febrile seizures, recurring in many illnesses and associated with a positive family history, are risk factors for later idiopathic generalized epilepsies.

Factors unrelated to prognosis are the type of infection, including whether or not there was an intracranial infection identified, and the EEG findings within 7 days of the onset.

Link with mesial temporal sclerosis

From pathological and pathophysiological viewpoints, there is a well-established link between prolonged, lateralized febrile seizures and later complex partial seizures of hippocampal origin. Initial suggestions that the seizure was the initiating event are currently being questioned. MRI evidence gives some support to the proposal that a prior abnormality in the temporal lobe leads to the lateralization of the seizure when the infant becomes febrile. Thus, mesial temporal sclerosis could be at least partially the result of a predisposition, although damage from the febrile seizure also seems to be important. No pathological correlations have been suggested for simple febrile seizures, but current investigations into the relationship between channelopathies and epilepsy may be illuminating.

Neurological development

The neurological status following an initial febrile seizure is unchanged from that prior to the seizure in 95 per cent of cases. In those who acquire new signs, hemipareses are most likely. Long-term EEG studies, with records taken serially over many months or years, may show age-dependent abnormalities such as centrotemporal spikes, which are not necessarily related to clinical expressions of seizures. Their relevance can be difficult to interpret.

Cognitive ability

Cognitive abilities are usually in line with those in the general population. In children admitted to hospital with febrile seizures, however, 5–15 per cent have global learning disorders and a further 12–19 per cent have specific reading difficulties. Attentional deficits are more common. Learning disorders occur most often in association with complex febrile seizures. Thus, both complex seizures and learning problems may reflect prior brain abnormalities. Aggressive outbursts, temper tantrums, unsociability and poor bladder and bowel control are all more frequent.

Social factors

The social implications of this condition should not be ignored. Febrile seizures occur in small children whose parents are likely to be young and inexperienced. When the first seizure occurs, most parents think that their child is dying. Subsequently, they spend more time watching their children at night or, if not watching, sleep poorly. Further seizures increase parental behavioural symptoms.

In summary, febrile seizures are for most children incidental events without serious sequelae. For some, the seizure is an alerting sign that long-term neurological problems may ensue. Full characterization at the initial presentation is essential.

DIFFERENTIAL DIAGNOSIS: NON-EPILEPTIC EVENTS

Non-epileptic events, which might be confused with seizures in this age group, are breath-holding spells, reflex anoxic attacks, hyperekplexia, benign paroxysmal vertigo, benign sleep myoclonus, benign infantile dystonia, benign paroxysmal torticollis and Meadow syndrome. Cardiac arrhythmias and syncope are rare. The features of these non-epileptic attacks are detailed in Chapter 4.

EPIDEMIOLOGY

Infancy is one of the peak times for the onset of seizures. This in part reflects the propensity for children to convulse in association with febrile illnesses during this age range, as considered above. Of infants with epilepsy, 29 per cent have benign partial epilepsy (Okumura *et al.*, 1996). Both benign and severe myoclonic epilepsies of infancy are extremely rare. Infantile spasms occur in between 24 and 42 children per 100 000 births but were found in 33 per cent of the cases of infantile epilepsy examined by Okumura *et al.* (1996).

SEIZURE TYPES AND EPILEPSIES

The epilepsies of infancy have been described in Chapter 3:

- benign partial epilepsy in infancy
- West syndrome
- benign myoclonic epilepsy of infancy
- severe myoclonic epilepsy of infancy.

Seizures in association with febrile illnesses have been given separate consideration above. They should be regarded as a sign of the potential development of epilepsy, even though, for most children, epilepsy does not supervene.

Cryptogenic localization-related epilepsy is a recognized entity but, with increasingly sophisticated imaging, is likely to be diagnosed less often.

Migrating partial seizures

A curiosity of infancy is a pattern of migrating partial seizures (Coppola *et al.*, 1995). The onset is before 6 months of age, with the peak between 2 and 4 months. The infants are previously normal. Then a few focal seizures occur over about 5 weeks, followed by more or less continuous partial attacks of apparently random origin involving both hemispheres. The ictal EEG is always the same, although its site of origin may differ. A rhythmic activity of decreasing frequency and increasing amplitude involves a larger and larger area during between 1 and 4 minutes. While very frequent seizures are present, there is a loss of acquired neurodevelopmental skills, and the growth of the head circumference ceases. In most cases, the seizures become less frequent after a few months, but some infants die. Gliosis of the hippocampus has been seen at post mortem.

AETIOLOGY

When seizures (not associated with fever) start in infancy and cannot be included in one of the epilepsy syndromes listed above, they are likely to be secondary to structural cerebral changes:

- **Neurocutaneous conditions** can be seen. It is important to examine the skin carefully when seizure disorders present early in life. Partial seizures may precede infantile spasms in tuberous sclerosis.
- **Major malformations** in conditions such as Aicardi syndrome, agyria/lissencephaly and hemi-megalencephaly may also present as partial seizures progressing to infantile spasms.
- **Pre-peduncular hamartoma** may begin as focal motor seizures before progressing to gelastic (laughing) attacks, the typical clinical manifestation.
- **Tumours**, including benign tumours, astrocytomas, gangliogliomas and dysembryoplastic neuroepithelial tumours, account for up to 2 per cent of infantile epilepsies.

- **Cortical dysplasias** are likely to be an underdiagnosed cause of infantile seizures.
- **Alpers' disease** is the only metabolic condition likely to present with partial seizures.
- **Prenatal, perinatal and immediate postnatal events** may also be followed by infantile seizures.

GENETICS

Details of the known genetic disorders in the major epilepsy syndromes in infancy are given in Chapter 5.

NEUROPHYSIOLOGICAL INVESTIGATIONS

The normal EEG shows a waking background rhythm of 1–3 Hz soon after birth, the frequency increasing with age so that by 12 months the predominant rhythm is 6 Hz. However, a considerable amount of both slower and faster rhythms is evident. *Tracé alternant* (*see* above) disappears by the age of 1 month.

The infant has sufficiently well-organized cerebral rhythms to produce epileptic spikes, but those seen in the occipital regions are not always associated with clinical seizures. EEG recording can be difficult in infancy, since cooperation may be very limited. Droperidol is first choice for sedation, if necessary, since it does not affect the EEG. A toddler will sometimes tolerate attachment of the electrodes for ambulatory monitoring better than those for a routine recording.

IMAGING

Structural imaging

Structural imaging, preferably with MRI, is indicated (as with epilepsies in any age group) for all infants with partial seizures, with the possible exception of febrile seizures. Nevertheless, if febrile seizures are associated with neurological abnormalities, even if these are transient, MRI may help with the understanding of the underlying pathology. There can be difficulties with the interpretation of scans in the very young. MRI depends partly on the ability to contrast myelinated white matter with cortex, but myelination is far from complete in infancy. Small areas of cortical dysplasia, or neuronal heterotopias, may be problematic, since the normal contrast with white matter is not fully defined. If seizures are persistent and not identified by early MRI, repeat imaging at a more mature age is indicated.

Functional imaging

Functional imaging is relevant in infants in whom a further delineation of the location of a lesion is required, especially if surgery is being considered.

Magnetic resonance spectroscopy

MR spectroscopy is likely to be used more frequently in future in the differentiation of ischaemic from infective lesions and in the non-invasive diagnosis of metabolic brain disorders.

MANAGEMENT

The choice of treatment for generalized tonic–clonic and partial seizures is as for other age groups. At the time of writing, lamotrigine, topiramate, oxcarbazepine, gabapentin, clobazam, tiagabine and piracetam have not been licensed in the UK for infants, i.e. children aged less than 2 years. Monotherapy with vigabatrin has been licensed only for infantile spasms. Special treatment issues in epilepsy syndromes are included in Chapters 3 and 6. It seems, however, important to re-emphasize that vigabatrin and carbamazepine are likely to make myoclonic seizures worse and that lamotrigine, although helpful in other myoclonia, exacerbates severe myoclonic epilepsy in infancy.

Formulation is an important issue. Infants do not, on the whole, take drugs readily. The pharmaceutical companies have made some efforts to produce child-friendly medicines and dispersible tablets. It is important for the prescriber to be acquainted with the strengths of liquid preparations and dispersible tablets as well as to instruct parents how to measure doses. Ease of measurement is essential, with the dose being rounded up or down so that the volume to be given is in millilitres rather than smaller divisions. Parents also need instruction in when to give another dose if the infant vomits, dribbles the medication out of the corner of the mouth, etc. If at least half the dose is lost within 20 minutes, it is usually appropriate for a further dose to be given.

PROGNOSIS

Further seizures/epilepsy

Apart from benign partial-onset seizures (either familial or non-familial), these diagnoses are often not apparent at onset, and epilepsy starting in infancy has a poor prognosis for freedom from seizures in the long term. This is largely a reflection of the high proportion of cases that occur secondary to structural lesions. These are considered under the separate headings for epilepsy syndromes (Chapter 3).

Cognitive implications

The cognitive implications are related mainly to the underlying cerebral disturbance of which the epilepsy is also a symptom. For West syndrome and severe myoclonic epilepsy in infancy, the cognitive outlook can be very poor. Approximately 90 per cent of those who have had infantile spasms have later learning difficulties, most being severely affected. All children with severe myoclonic epilepsy have significant problems. Although those with benign myoclonic epilepsy were originally reported to be of normal intelligence, specific disabilities such as dyspraxia and dyslexia often cause educational difficulties.

SOCIAL FACTORS

Not only are epileptic seizures very frightening for the parents to witness, but they also bring with them fears about subsequent physical and mental handicap. Many of these fears are realistic, and it is important for the paediatrician to categorize the child's seizure disorder correctly, so that any information given is as accurate as possible.

Coming to terms with a child's continuing neurological disability is a difficult process for the parents. Anxiety about the child may restrict baby-sitting opportunities, attendance at mother and baby groups etc., with a resultant reduction in the number of opportunities for social contact for both parent and infant. Emphasis on the needs relating to the supervision of the infant with epilepsy can cause other siblings to have reduced interaction with their parents, with consequent feelings of neglect.

Seizures in children (2 years to pre-puberty)

DIFFERENTIAL DIAGNOSIS

Breath-holding spells, reflex anoxic attacks and benign paroxysmal vertigo are less common than in infants and tend to disappear completely by the age of 4 years. Vasovagal attacks and, less commonly, cardiac arrhythmias are the most probable cause of diagnostic confusion in older children. Narcolepsy/cataplexy or episodic ataxias may commence as early as 2 years of age. As puberty approaches, non-epileptic attack disorder ('pseudoseizures') can cause confusion; sexual abuse should always be considered in these cases.

EPIDEMIOLOGY

Epilepsy is prevalent in about 5 to 10 per 1000 children of school age. Those with cerebral palsy and those with learning difficulties show a much higher rate, variously estimated to lie between 20 and 40 per cent. The lower the intelligence, the more likely is epilepsy also to be present. The prevalances and syndrome descriptions of the epilepsy syndromes that start in this age range are given in Chapter 3.

SEIZURE TYPES AND EPILEPSIES

All seizure types may be seen in this age period:

- **Myoclonia of early onset**, i.e. presenting before the age of 10 years, is likely to be of more serious import for learning and for continuing epilepsy than that presenting later. Myoclonia presenting after the age of 10 years most frequently heralds the onset of juvenile myoclonic epilepsy.
- **Absences of early onset**, i.e. before the age of 4 or 5 years, are also a cause for greater concern compared with those of onset beyond the age of 5. They are more likely to be associated with myoclonia, thus being more difficult to control, and to have a greater risk of epilepsy continuing into adulthood.
- **Idiopathic generalized epilepsies** are most likely to commence in this age range.
- **Idiopathic localization-related epilepsies.** It is important to be acquainted with the characteristics of the benign partial epilepsies (*see* Chapter 3) for a correct characterization of epilepsy in the first decade.
- **Symptomatic epilepsies.** At least 40 per cent of children with epilepsy in middle childhood have partial-onset seizures, with or without secondary generalization, which are symptomatic of structural lesions.
- **Other epilepsies.** Further details of myoclonic astatic epilepsy, Lennox–Gastaut syndrome, the various types of epilepsy associated with absences, those with partial symptomatology and juvenile myoclonic epilepsy can be found in Chapter 3.

At no other time in the life of someone who has epilepsy is the condition so likely to be temporary. Not only are several epilepsy types most likely to start at this age, but it is also towards the end of this period that benign partial epilepsies, in particular benign epilepsy of childhood with centrotemporal spikes, tend to remit.

AETIOLOGY

Symptomatic epilepsies tend to be relatively less prevalent at this age than in neonates and infants. It is nevertheless important to search assiduously for structural lesions in children whose clinical or EEG features are not typical of a benign type of epilepsy.

- **Inborn errors of metabolism** are unlikely to present *de novo* with seizures after 2 years of age, but this remote possibility should not be ignored.
- **Acquired causes** of hypoglycaemia, porphyria or neurodegenerative disease should not be forgotten.
- **New structural lesions,** for example tumours, acute vascular events, scarring from previous infections and head injuries, are more common than in young infants.
- **Cortical dysplasia** is determined before the twentieth week of gestation, but the associated symptomatic seizures may not start until well into childhood.

Idiopathic epilepsies usually begin in middle to late childhood.

GENETICS

The genetic implications of those epilepsies with a known genetic basis are given in Chapter 3, along with descriptions of the individual syndromes:

- **Idiopathic generalized epilepsies**, even if they do not have a defined gene location, are recognized as being, at least to some extent, genetically determined. For many, however, the inheritance is considered to be complex.
- **Idiopathic localization-related epilepsies.** Benign partial epilepsies are also, as a whole, considered to be genetically determined. However, benign epilepsy with centrotemporal spikes is the only one in which the gene has been identified.
- **Symptomatic epilepsies.** Of more practical importance in this age range is the recognition of potentially inheritable generalized conditions of which seizures are an early sign. Late infantile neuronal ceroid lipofuscinosis is an important, albeit rare, example. Tuberous sclerosis and other neurocutaneous syndromes may be highlighted by the onset of seizures after the age of 2 years. Correct identification of such aetiologies clearly allows informed genetic counselling.

NEUROPHYSIOLOGICAL INVESTIGATIONS

With increasing age, cooperation with EEG recording is likely to improve, although for learning disabled children and those with behavioural difficulties, problems with obtaining artefact-free records may persist. Droperidol is the most suitable sedative, if necessary. A brief summary of EEG findings in various neurodegenerative disorders can be found in Wallace (1996), a more detailed description being available in Naidu and Niedermeyer (1993).

The normal EEG

Age-related changes

On the EEG, the background frequencies continue to increase with age, with theta rhythms (5–7 Hz) predominating in middle childhood and a gradual acceleration to alpha rhythms (8–2 Hz) towards puberty. Records indistinguishable from those of adults are expected by 12–14 years of age.

Hyperventilation

Young children find it difficult to cooperate with hyperventilation, but unless learning disabled or behaviourally disturbed, most will overbreathe, when required, after the age of 4 or 5 years. Before the age of about 10 years, particularly in the younger children, there is a reduction in the frequency and an increase in the amplitude of activity during hyperventilation. This leads to a domination, for the period of the test, of high-voltage slow activity. Hyperventilation is particularly useful for the precipitation of the regular 3 Hz spike-and-wave characteristically seen in childhood absence seizures. It may, however, precipitate other types of seizure discharge.

Photosensitivity

Photosensitivity becomes more common with increasing age throughout childhood. Apart from its presence in severe myoclonic epilepsy in infants, it always suggests an idiopathic generalized epilepsy, thus having genetic implications. In late infantile neuronal ceroid lipofuscinosis, characteristic posterior spike discharges are seen when the child is looking at a light that is flashing slowly; the spikes disappear at high flash frequencies or if the child looks away from the light.

EEG and seizures

The EEG is highly likely to be abnormal in true epileptic seizures, but even ictal recordings can be unhelpful if the discharges emanate from a deep structure such as the inferior frontal or mesial temporal area. In addition, seizures starting in these areas are those most likely to be associated with changes in behaviour. Nevertheless, if many attacks are occurring without an associated EEG change (even after activating procedures such as hyperventilation, photic stimulation, sleep deprivation and sleep itself), non-epileptic attack disorders should be suspected.

Surgery for epilepsy

This is more likely to be considered in this age range than in those younger. Invasive recording with foramen ovale or strip or grid electrodes may be poorly tolerated unless sedation is given. In these circumstances, the sedative must be chosen with care so that seizure discharges are not unnecessarily suppressed.

Other neurophysiological investigations

Other investigations, such as visual evoked potentials, electroretinograms, nerve conduction studies and electromyography, can be helpful in the diagnoses of underlying conditions, particularly when a degenerative disorder of the nervous system is suspected. Magnetoencephalography is still limited to a few centres; it requires the patient to be absolutely immobile.

IMAGING

Indication

- **Partial seizures.** Cerebral imaging is required for children presenting with seizures of partial onset. However, if the clinical and EEG features are absolutely characteristic of benign epilepsy with centrotemporal spikes, imaging is not required. If there are any doubts about this diagnosis, it is safer to request a scan.
- **Generalized seizures.** If seizures are confidently considered to be primary generalized, i.e. idiopathic, in nature, imaging is not required. Thus, imaging is not necessary for childhood or adolescent absence epilepsies, generalized tonic-clonic seizures on awakening, and juvenile myoclonic epilepsy.

Method

MR imaging is preferred. After the age of 2 years, myelination, albeit not complete, is sufficiently advanced for good differentiation between grey and white matter to be expected. This differentiation may be somewhat obscured in areas where cortical dysplasia is demonstrated. In addition to demonstrating structural changes that may be dysplastic, vascular, infective, neoplastic or traumatic in origin, MRI can be specifically helpful in the diagnosis of degenerative disorders that present with seizures.

CT scanning can show some relevant changes but does not give the same definition of cortical structures as MR. Intracerebral calcification can be seen on CT but not MR images.

Magnetic resonance spectroscopy can be used to identify epileptogenic disorders in which cerebral chemistry changes occur locally or generally. Proton (^{1}H) spectroscopy allows the determination of brain lactate level, which may be raised in epilepsies associated with mitochondrial disorders. ^{31}Phosphate MRS gives indications of local high-energy phosphate levels and can be used to confirm lateralization in temporal lobe epilepsy, in which the affected side has a reduced phosphocreatine:inorganic phosphate ratio.

Positron emission tomography is not widely available but may be used for the interictal localization of seizure foci by non-invasive means. Its main application is in presurgical work-up.

Single photon emission tomography, although more readily available than PET, is more difficult to use to greatest effect. Again, it is most applicable for children being investigated with a view to surgery. Ideally, ictal and interictal images should be obtained so that a comparison may be made between them. For the ictal records, the isotope must be injected absolutely at the start of the seizure: this is the major disadvantage of this type of imaging and a particular problem if there is no aura or only a brief event (e.g. in frontal lobe seizures).

MANAGEMENT

Anti-epileptic medication

Dosing frequency

Younger children generally metabolize drugs more quickly than those who are older. Thus, for medications with a relatively short half-life, such as carbamazepine, three times daily dosing may be necessary to ensure an adequate level throughout the 24 hours. Slow-release formulations are almost invariably produced as tablets, so their use in small children can be problematical. As the child grows and activities outside the home increase, the timing of drug administration should, if possible, be reduced to twice a day. If suitable, drugs with a long half-life are preferred since once daily dosing is then allowable.

Formulation

Formulation remains important. Even those of 10 years and over may refuse to swallow tablets. Cooperation with taking medication can be particularly difficult to ensure in this age range, particularly in older and larger patients with learning difficulties.

Choice of medication

The choice of anti-epileptic treatment remains dependent on the seizure type or syndrome (Wallace, 2000), rather more therapies being available for this age range than for infants. Licences in the UK have been given for gabapentin and oxcarbazepine for those over 6 years; lamotrigine and topiramate for all children in this age range; clobazam for 3-year-olds and above; and tiagabine for those of 12 years and older. Piracetam is not officially recommended for patients under the age of 16 years, but it can be helpful for myoclonia resistant to other therapies.

It cannot be overemphasized that both carbamazepine and vigabatrin can make myoclonic and atonic seizures worse and neither is effective for absence seizures. Gabapentin may also precipitate myoclonia.

Compliance

Treatment does not stop at the prescription of drugs. Explanations about the therapy and suggestions related to ensuring compliance and the importance of regular dosing, with due regard to the way of life of individual families, are part of treatment.

Complex epilepsy

Only about 80 per cent of children with epilepsy will become completely seizure free on what appears to be optimal medication. In particular, children with severe mental and physical disability respond poorly. Furthermore, for a substantial minority, epilepsy is only one of the child's neurological disabilities.

Practical approach

It is important to have a realistic approach. Atypical absences and myoclonic jerks may be accepted in children who have severe physical handicaps and are not independently mobile, but such attacks can in themselves be dangerous in the more physically competent. Strenuous attempts should be made to eliminate all typical absence seizures and all generalized tonic-clonic seizures occurring during the daytime in children attending mainstream schools. On the other hand, it may be impossible to control all the seizures of those with the Lennox–Gastaut syndrome and other severe epilepsies without producing unacceptable side effects. Only by a correct characterization of the epilepsy and by a good knowledge of the advantages and limitations of the treatments available will optimal treatment be achieved.

Surgery

Middle to late childhood is probably the best time for considering surgery. It might be considered for children with localization-related epilepsies secondary to defined non-progressive structural abnormalities. Surgery for epilepsy is considered in more detail in Chapter 6, as are vagus nerve stimulation and dietary therapies.

PROGNOSIS

With regard to prognosis for further seizures, childhood epilepsies can be broadly divided into three groups:

1. **Self-limiting epilepsies** are unlikely to persist into adulthood. These include childhood absence epilepsy, benign epilepsy of childhood with centrotemporal spikes, and benign early-onset and late-onset occipital epilepsies.
2. **Idiopathic generalized epilepsies** often persist into adulthood. This group is dominated by juvenile myoclonic epilepsy and other epilepsies associated with photosensitivity and/or primary generalized tonic-clonic seizures. Treatment is likely to be needed for life. However, this group, on

the whole, responds well to appropriate therapy, usually valproate or lamotrigine.

3. **Epilepsies with permanent structural or physical abnormalities** comprise epilepsies secondary to cortical dysplasias and other definable structural changes, Lennox–Gastaut syndrome, myoclonic–astatic epilepsy, variants of absence epilepsies and severe epilepsies persisting from infancy; seizures are very likely to continue.

COGNITIVE IMPLICATIONS

Cognitive prognosis

Cognitive abilities are difficult to assess in a predictive manner in infancy. After the age of 2 years, learning difficulties, whether specific or global, are easier to recognize and define. Some epilepsies, such as Lennox–Gastaut syndrome and some syndromes in which epilepsy is common, for example Rett syndrome (*see* Chapter 4), are invariably associated with severe learning disability. When a child presents with seizures, it is important to consider whether these are secondary to a condition in which cognitive problems co-exist.

Epilepsies with cognitive symptomatology

Epilepsies whose symptomatologies are largely cognitive have been described in Chapter 3. Conventionally, they are the Landau–Kleffner syndrome and epilepsy with continuous spike-waves during slow wave sleep. However, atypical absences in association with any epilepsy lead to lapses in awareness, as do classical childhood absences. Rarely, severe forms of benign epilepsy with centrotemporal spikes can merge into Landau–Kleffner syndrome.

Simultaneous cognitive and EEG testing shows that a transient impairment of cognition occurs in association with spike discharges. It is very rare for intellectual deterioration to be secondary to epilepsy itself, but a standstill in cognitive and educational progress can accompany severe epilepsies.

Effect of medication

Anti-epileptic drugs, given at conventional therapeutic dosages, do not, on the whole, interfere with cognitive processes. By reducing the number of seizure discharges, their actions are more likely to improve continuous attention and allow a more consistent input of information. Higher dosages may, however, lead to drowsiness, and it is important that a sensible balance is achieved between efficacy and adverse effects.

Schooling

Most children with epilepsy attend mainstream schools, but underachievement is more common than expected. A further consideration of schooling is given in Chapter 9.

SOCIAL FACTORS

Epilepsy is likely to produce socially limiting factors in all age ranges. The social stigma of having epilepsy is considered here in more detail.

Nursery care

In the preschool child, attendance at mother-and-toddler groups may be curtailed by the mother's fear that her child will have a seizure in front of other mothers, and by difficulties with fitting educational and social activities into a schedule full of clinic appointments. Later, nursery placement can be problematic because of the potential need for emergency treatment, such as rectal diazepam, with its attendant issues relating to special training and child protection. Children who are not able to attend neighbourhood nurseries or school, and/or are taken to educational placements in special transport, miss normal social contact, and their parents do not meet those of children living close by.

Lack of independence

The parents of children with epilepsy, understandably, find it difficult to allow their children to gain the independence that would be usual with increasing age. Those at risk of sleep-associated seizures often sleep in their parents' bed well into late childhood. Letting go becomes more difficult as adolescence approaches and peers without epilepsy go out on their bicycles, take the bus into town, play in amusement arcades or go to the local swimming pool. Children who have classical childhood absence epilepsy and those who have very frequent spike discharges are clearly at risk if riding a bicycle on the main road, but there is no increased risk for those whose seizures are entirely nocturnal or occur only on awakening. Once again, the correct categorization of seizure type and epilepsy syndrome is essential in management. When swimming, it is recommended that any child who has epilepsy be accompanied by an adult who has one-to-one responsibility for that child and who is in the water with the child.

Managing medication

Responsibility for compliance with medication passes from parent to child with age. Most teenagers of normal ability should be able to manage their own medication, but attempts to achieve this before the age of about 12 years are usually unsuccessful. Household regimes often make the complete regularity of treatment difficult: when both parents are working outside the home, and at different times of day, there is often a poorly defined system for the regular administration of drugs, neither parent knowing whether or not medication has been given and therefore not administering it for fear of overdosing. Some children develop strategies for hiding tablets, for example in the cushions on the settee or behind the refrigerator, even when the drug is 'given' to them; parents are often ashamed of these activities and deny that they occur.

Epilepsy in teenagers

Even for healthy teenagers, coping with emerging adulthood is a major challenge. A chronic disability such as epilepsy simply magnifies the problems of adolescence. Epilepsy and its medications have a direct bearing on several major aspects of lifestyle, such as education and employment prospects, driving ability, the use of alcohol and recreational drugs, relationships, contraception, pregnancy and parenthood. Education is at a critical stage, and employment prospects are just being realized. Self-consciousness is paramount, and deviations from peer group norms assume great importance for the adolescent. Thus, epilepsy can be disastrous for self-esteem and self-identity (Appleton *et al.*, 1997; Smith, 1998).

PSYCHOSOCIAL FACTORS

Epilepsy at any age is associated with a risk of psychosocial handicap, and especially so in the adolescent. Epilepsy restricts a teenager's independence, impedes the development of a normal identity and sexuality, and presents a barrier to normal relationships. Having seizures and needing to take medication is embarrassing and socially limiting, and may permanently dent a young person's self-esteem. Social interaction is further damaged by the anxiety and depression that commonly accompany epilepsy. Low self-esteem and social isolation lead to a poor development of social skills and increased anxiety, in a vicious circle. Pressures exerted by parental anxiety and, more importantly, by peers also shape the behaviour of the teenager with epilepsy.

Patient anxiety
Patients with epilepsy have many anxieties, which are often poorly expressed. These include the fear of having a seizure in public, of causing self-injury and of receiving a hostile reaction from others should they have a seizure. A consequent avoidance of social situations may further lower self-esteem.

Parental anxiety and pressure
Epilepsy in an individual affects the whole family. The attitudes of parents, family and, above all, peers to the epilepsy will strongly influence the response of the teenager. The teenager with disability is more likely to be treated by his or her family and elders as a child than as an adult. Two main factors contribute.

    Restrictions imposed by concerned parents, suggested by peers or initiated by the patient are often unnecessary or inappropriate and may be very damaging, denying the opportunity for friendship and encouraging social isolation. Leisure pursuits are very important in the teenage years for building normal relationships. The overprotected teenager easily becomes overdependent upon parents and peers.

Parents may have **lowered expectations** and aspirations for a child or teenager with epilepsy; this can become a damaging, self-fulfilling prophecy since the parents' attitude may diminish a teenager's self-esteem and lead to poor performance. Epilepsy itself is not an excuse for underachievement.

Peer pressure

The teenage years bring an intense peer pressure not to be different. For the teenager with epilepsy, this has important implications:

- **Treatment compliance** may be poor since the tablets remind teenagers that they are different.
- **Lack of openness.** Teenagers may be unwilling to discuss problems and fears about their epilepsy.
- **Seizure-provoking activity.** Teenagers are likely to come under pressure to participate in behaviours that may potentially provoke seizures, for example sleep deprivation, alcohol, recreational drugs and exposure to flashing lights.

MANAGEMENT

In managing the adolescent patient with epilepsy, the emphasis must, as always, be placed upon a correct diagnosis, the appropriate use of anti-epileptic medication and encouraging treatment compliance. In adolescence, there are additional important areas of management including the provision of information about epilepsy and its implications for lifestyle, aiming to maintain independence and to tackle the psychosocial consequences of epilepsy.

DIAGNOSIS

A correct diagnosis of the cause of blackouts is, perhaps more than at any other age, essential in young people. The consequences of a misdiagnosis of epilepsy may be disastrous in terms of impaired education, employment and driving prospects, unnecessary medication and diminished self-esteem. Important issues surround epilepsy diagnosis in the teenage years.

Epilepsies that present first in adolescence

Juvenile myoclonic epilepsy is the most important example since this condition is underdiagnosed yet carries specific clinical management implications. A diagnosis of juvenile myoclonic epilepsy implies the need for a long-term prescription of sodium valproate (as well as folate in females in view of potential teratogenicity) and careful attention to lifestyle, including a regular sleep pattern and minimizing alcohol intake. Photosensitivity, either in isolation or as part of an epilepsy syndrome, may also first appear in adolescence. Less common epilepsies presenting typically at this age include juvenile absence epilepsy, generalized tonic-clonic seizures on awakening and late-onset benign occipital epilepsy.

Epilepsies that improve during adolescence

Childhood-onset epilepsies may occasionally remit during the teenage years. Benign childhood epilepsy with centrotemporal spikes, for example, almost always remits at puberty. Teenagers with the typical previous history of sleep-provoked simple partial seizures involving the face and arm, and a typical EEG, can be reassured that medication can be safely discontinued without significant risk of recurrence.

Blackouts that mimic epilepsy in adolescence

Blackouts commonly mistaken for seizures in this age group include conditions that commonly present for the first time in the teenage years, for example vasovagal syncope, psychogenic non-epileptic attack disorder and migraine.

MEDICATION AND COMPLIANCE

Which medication?

Although the principles of use of anti-epileptic medications are identical to those in any age group, it is particularly important to ensure that the type and dose of treatment are appropriate in teenagers. The type of epilepsy, as well as the effectiveness and tolerability of the treatment itself, determines the choice of medication. The general principle is to use the lowest effective dose of a medication with few side effects in a once or twice daily dose.

Side effects

The **cognitive side effects** of anti-epileptic medications are important at any age, but in childhood and adolescence, even mild cognitive dysfunction may permanently harm educational and employment prospects.

Cosmetic effects of phenytoin make this drug a poor choice for the first-line treatment of young people, particularly young women. Weight gain is sometimes a prominent side effect of valproate, and this may limit its usefulness in weight-conscious young people.

Young women taking enzyme-inducing anti-epileptic medications (e.g. carbamazepine, phenytoin, oxcarbazepine and topiramate) must be warned of their interaction with the **oral contraceptive pill**.

All females of child-bearing potential taking medication need to understand the potential **teratogenic risk**. There is some evidence that folate reduces this risk for enzyme-inducing anti-epileptic medications and valproate. A pharmacological dose of folate 5 mg daily thus seems a sensible addition to any anti-epileptic medication, with the knowledge that at least 30 per cent of teenage pregnancies are unplanned.

Compliance

Poor compliance with anti-epileptic medication occurs at all ages owing to several factors:

- a **denial** of the epilepsy;
- **medication side effects**, including possible teratogenicity;
- **complacency** with regard to good seizure control, paradoxically resulting in poor compliance and seizure recurrence.

Additional factors lead to poor compliance in the teenager with epilepsy:

- **peer pressure** not to be different, each dose of tablets being a reminder that they are different;
- **rebellion** against parental involvement in the management of their epilepsy.

Lifestyle

Epilepsy has lifestyle implications that are of particular concern to the teenager. The teenager is likely to be at a crucial stage in school education or just beginning employment or career training (*see* Chapter 9). Epilepsy can make a major adverse impact upon educational and employment success; career choices are inevitably restricted by the diagnosis of epilepsy. Issues such as driving, the use of alcohol and recreational drugs, and the pursuit of sport and leisure activities, travel, the use of VDUs and exposure to flashing disco lights are all-important topics to raise with the teenager. It is particularly important to address the issues of relationships, contraception and pregnancy.

Advice on lifestyle, including cooking, swimming, bathing, open fires and childcare, is applicable to anyone with epilepsy. The general principles upon which lifestyle advice is based are as follows:

- education in terms of the risks presented by epilepsy, while encouraging teenagers to make their own decisions about risk avoidance;
- acknowledging that living with epilepsy is about living with certain risks;
- accepting the legal ban on driving, with its consequences for certain career choices.

Driving

It is essential that young people are informed of the driving laws (*see* Chapter 9). Adolescents may, through ill-informed discussion with their peers, hold misplaced beliefs about the legal driving restrictions or not understand that their epilepsy medication does not prevent them from holding a driving licence.

Alcohol and drugs

The majority of teenagers consume occasional alcohol, and a significant proportion experiment with illegal substances. Aside from the legal issues, there are several reasons why alcohol is detrimental to epilepsy control and these are discussed later (*see* Chapter 9).

Sport and leisure

This is an important issue for any young person. Although some limitation of certain leisure pursuits is often appropriate, undue restriction may have major psychosocial consequences. A sensible balance must be achieved with the teenager's agreement. In general, restrictions must be kept to a minimum.

Other issues

Missing sleep may provoke seizures in vulnerable individuals such as those with idiopathic generalized epilepsy. Those known to be photosensitive on EEG testing should be advised to be cautious at discos and when using computer screens. A more common problem, however, is that teenagers, parents or teachers believe that the individual should avoid flashing lights and VDU screens simply because of the diagnosis of epilepsy. It is therefore important also to inform patients who are not photosensitive.

The consultation

Teenagers often find attendance at the paediatric clinic embarrassing and inappropriate. The physician caring for teenagers with epilepsy should aim for the following:

- See the teenager in a clinic with other teenagers or adults.
- Direct the consultation to the teenager rather than to the parents. For example, invite the teenager to introduce his or her parents or carers.
- Discuss adult topics such as driving, pregnancy and alcohol with the teenager.
- Speak to the teenager alone during the consultation; an opportunity arises if the physical examination is being conducted in another room.
- Involve other team members. Consider giving the opportunity to speak to an epilepsy specialist nurse or voluntary field worker; like many adults, teenagers often open up to a nurse or lay volunteer more than to a doctor.

- Offer written material on the relevant aspects of epilepsy.
- Encourage responsibility. Carers should allow teenagers appropriate responsibility, for example for their own tablets, and help them to gain independence.
- Prescribe user-friendly medications. This involves choosing medication appropriate for the type of epilepsy, with few side effects, that is required to be taken only once or twice daily (thus avoiding taking tablets to school or work).

CONCLUSION

The challenge of adolescence is compounded by disabilities such as epilepsy. The problems faced by teenagers with epilepsy are not unique to them but apply, often to a lesser extent, across the spectrum of patients with epilepsy. Epilepsy can be harmful to personal and social development, as well as directly impacting upon driving ability, alcohol use, pregnancy and contraception. The physician must encourage an adult approach to teenage epilepsy management, thereby giving the best opportunity for patients to cope with their disability and comply with treatment.

Epilepsy and women

Several issues concerning epilepsy and its treatment predominantly or exclusively affect women. These fall into the following categories:

- periods and fertility
- pill
- pregnancy
- parenthood

Issues such as the cosmetic and osteoporotic effects of anti-epileptic drugs are also predominantly female issues.

PERIODS AND FERTILITY

The menstrual cycle

Seizures are often reported to cluster around the menstrual period (catamenial epilepsy), although when studied prospectively (Duncan *et al.*, 1993), this is found in only about 5 per cent of women. In humans, the amount of 'epileptiform' activity on the interictal EEG is increased by oestrogen and decreased by progesterone. In animal models, oestrogen is proconvulsive, enhancing neuronal excitability, whereas progesterone is relatively anti-convulsive. The contribution of premenstrual syndrome and fluid retention to seizure frequency is unknown.

Specific attempts to treat catamenial seizures have shown mixed results. Progesterone treatment is well tolerated and is worth considering as additional therapy in women with a clear catamenial pattern (Herzog, 1995), although it may cause reversible dose-related fatigue and depression in a minority. It must be remembered that the progesterone-only pill, when used alone, is unreliable as an oral contraceptive. Acetazolamide, a weak anti-epileptic with diuretic effects, is relatively ineffective. The dramatic improvements reported with intermittent clobazam (Feely *et al.*, 1982), dosing only on the days around the menstrual cycle, are often disappointing in practice.

Fertility

Women with epilepsy show reduced fertility, perhaps to about 60 per cent that of the general population (Schupf and Ottoman, 1994). This is attributable to several factors:

- decision not to have children;
- reduced libido through a fear of seizures or medication side effects;
- menstrual and reproductive endocrine disorders, including a lowered level of sex hormone-binding globulin in patients on enzyme-inducing anti-epileptic medications, an increased number of anovulatory cycles (Cummings *et al.*, 1995) and abnormalities of ovarian structure and function in women with epilepsy, particularly those taking valproate or carbamazepine (Isojarvi *et al.*, 1993).

THE CONTRACEPTIVE PILL AND HORMONE REPLACEMENT THERAPY

Oral contraceptive pill

Although oestrogen is potentially proconvulsant, oral contraception usually has no adverse effect upon epilepsy. Nevertheless, it should be prescribed with caution in patients with severe epilepsy or those with a history of status epilepticus.

Contraception failure can result from the enhanced metabolism of ethinyl-oestradiol and levonorgestrel following treatment with enzyme-inducing anti-epileptic medications such as carbamazepine, oxcarbazepine, phenytoin, phenobarbitone and topiramate. The failure rate (50 µg pill) increases from 0.7 to 3.1 per 100 woman years while on enzyme inducers (Mattson *et al.*, 1986), being likely to be even higher with the more widely prescribed 'Minipill' (35 µg of oestrogen or less). Women using the pill for contraception should therefore take a preparation containing at least 50 µg oestrogen;

doses of up to 100 µg daily may be necessary to prevent breakthrough bleeding, a clear sign of an inadequate oestrogen level. Even so, it is sensible to advise alternative methods of contraception if taking enzyme-inducing anti-epileptic medications. One way of reducing the risk of ovulation when on enzyme inducers (especially phenytoin) is to advise the patient to take three consecutive contraceptive pill packs followed by a 4-day break.

The progesterone-only pill is even less reliable than the combined pill for people on enzyme-inducing drugs. This is because the breakthrough bleeding that is normal with the progesterone-only pill cannot be distinguished from anticonvulsant-induced contraception failure. Depot progesterone injections are associated with water retention; this may, in theory, aggravate the epilepsy.

Anti-epileptic medications not associated with induction of the relevant liver enzymes (valproate, lamotrigine, gabapentin, tiagabine and vigabatrin) do not cause oral contraceptive failure.

Hormone replacement therapy

Being a replacement rather than an addition, hormone replacement therapy does not significantly influence epilepsy, but patients taking liver enzyme inducers will still need a larger oestrogen dose. Hormone replacement therapy may be best prescribed as patches rather than tablets in these circumstances since this overcomes the first-pass effect in the liver.

PREGNANCY

Although, in general, women with epilepsy tend to have fewer children than those without, about 1 in 200 pregnant women have epilepsy. There are three main problem areas:

- the **effect of pregnancy on the epilepsy** (mainly its effects on anti-epileptic drugs);
- the **effect of epilepsy on the pregnancy**;
- the **effect of anti-epileptic medication** on the unborn child (teratogenicity).

Effect of pregnancy on epilepsy

About a third of patients show a deterioration in seizure control during pregnancy. This can often be attributed to poor drug compliance or an inappropriate reduction in the prescribed medication by patient or doctor through a fear of adverse fetal effects from the anti-epileptic medication. The situation may be compounded by vomiting and poor sleep. Changes in anti-epileptic medication pharmacokinetics (Yerby *et al.*, 1990) – volume of distribution, hepatic metabolism and renal clearance – reduce the serum level of some drugs. The protein binding of some anti-epileptic medications is reduced owing to increased competition by sex steroid hormones for the available protein binding sites and by a lowered serum albumin level.

Overall, the effect of pregnancy on the epilepsy is not too troublesome. An episode of status epilepticus complicates fewer than 1 per cent of pregnancies, and major seizures complicate labour in 1–2 per cent of cases (Donaldson, 1989).

Effect of epilepsy on pregnancy

Simple partial, complex partial, myoclonic and absence seizures are not considered harmful to the fetus. Generalized tonic-clonic seizures, particularly during status epilepticus, may, in theory, lead to sufficient hypoxaemia to harm the baby. There is, however, no evidence to support this. The major hazard to the fetus from an epileptic seizure is through direct trauma to the abdomen during a seizure.

Effect of anti-epileptic medication

Teratogenicity in humans has been established with the four conventional anti-epileptic medications: valproate, carbamazepine, phenytoin and phenobarbitone. Topiramate is teratogenic in rats, but there are grounds to believe that this is a species-specific effect related to its carbonic anhydrase inhibitor action (*see* Chapter 6); there is no evidence that topiramate is harmful to the human fetus. The teratogenic potential of the other new agents (gabapentin, lamotrigine, levetiracetam, oxcarbazepine, tiagabine and vigabatrin) is also unknown, although animal studies and the limited evidence so far from humans have suggested them to be of lower risk than conventional medication.

Of the infants born to mothers with epilepsy, minor malformations are seen in 6–20 per cent and major malformations affect 4–6 per cent (Gaily and Granstrom, 1992). This represents approximately a doubling of the risk compared with babies of mothers not taking anti-epileptic medication.

It is important to emphasize two points to potential mothers with epilepsy:

- Up to 90 per cent of infants exposed to anticonvulsants *in utero* will be entirely normal.
- Major birth defects occur in 3 per cent of pregnancies independently of any drug exposure or genetic history.

Minor malformations associated with conventional anti-epileptic medications include hypertelorism, epicanthic folds, deficient nasal growth, abnormal ears, a low hairline, distal digital and nail hypoplasia and altered finger-tip dermatoglyphic patterns. Many of these changes are outgrown in the first few years of life (Koch *et al.*, 1992). The association of these changes with medication has been questioned since such features were seen in children born to mothers with epilepsy before the introduction of anti-epileptic medications – a maternal genetic influence responsible for both the epilepsy and the epicanthic and digital hypoplasia has been proposed (Gaily and Granstrom, 1992).

Major malformations are associated particularly with phenytoin and phenobarbitone, and include cleft lip and palate (five times the normal risk) and congenital heart disease (a fourfold increase in risk). The risk of neural tube defect increases from a background rate of about 0.2 per cent to 1–2 per cent in mothers taking valproate (Omtzigt *et al.*, 1992) and 0.9 per cent in mothers taking carbamazepine (Rosa, 1991).

Folate and the prevention of teratogenicity

In an effort to reduce the risk of neural tube defects in the developing fetus, a folate supplement (5 mg daily) is widely recommended for women on anti-epileptic medications who might become pregnant. A low serum folate level is associated with an increased risk of fetal abnormality and spontaneous abortion. Impaired folate activity is likely to be a major cause of the teratogenicity related to anti-epileptic medication. Serum folate is reduced in the majority of patients receiving enzyme-inducing anti-epileptic medications.

Valproate does not induce liver enzymes but does interfere with folate metabolism. The newer drugs gabapentin, vigabatrin and lamotrigine (notwithstanding lamotrigine's weak anti-folate properties *in vitro*) do not affect the serum folate level. A study of valproate-induced neural tube defects in mice showed a significant benefit from folate supplementation (Elmazar *et al.*, 1992). A dramatic reduction (72 per cent) in the number of fetal neural tube defects in the infants of (non-epileptic) mothers with a previous spina bifida pregnancy was seen following folate 4 mg daily prescribed from before conception (MRC, 1991b). Other major malformations (although not cleft lip or palate) have also been reduced by periconceptual folate supplements.

Thus, all women on anti-epileptic medication who are not actively using contraception should be advised also to take a 5 mg daily folate supplement.

Management of pregnancy in women with epilepsy

Consensus management guidelines concerning women with epilepsy who plan a pregnancy have been published (Delgado-Escueta and Janz, 1992; Crawford *et al.*, 1999).

General points

The goal of treating seizures in a woman of child-bearing potential is to optimize seizure control while minimizing fetal risk. The teratogenic potential of anti-epileptic medications is naturally of great concern to women planning a pregnancy, and all medication is potentially harmful to early fetal development. It is important to provide accurate and patient-centred information on the known risks to women with epilepsy who are planning a pregnancy.

Before conception

The patient and physician should each ask themselves, 'Is the anti-epileptic medication necessary?' A review of anti-epileptic medication before conception is important for all potentially reproductive women with epilepsy. Once a woman is aware that she is pregnant, it is often too late to prevent drug-related teratogenicity. A patient free from seizures for 2–3 years may wish to attempt a withdrawal of medication before conception, balancing the risk to her fetus against the risks to herself, her lifestyle and her driving licence that a further seizure might bring (*see* Chapter 6).

If anti-epileptic medication cannot be stopped (which is usually the case), it is important that the preconception treatment regimen is modified in order to minimize the risk of teratogenicity.

- Give **information** about the potential teratogenicity of individual drugs (*see* Fig. 8.1, p. 222, and Chapter 6).
- Consider **alternative medication** that may be less harmful to the fetus; for example, change sodium valproate to lamotrigine (although firm evidence of the teratogenic potential of lamotrigine is presently lacking).
- Use a **single drug at the lowest effective dose**. The risk of teratogenicity is greater at higher doses and with multiple medications.
- Use **slow-release formulations** (e.g. of carbamazepine or valproate) and space the doses out to three or four times daily to avoid unnecessary peak plasma levels.
- Prescribe **folate** 5 mg daily for 3 months before conception and during the first trimester (as well as throughout pregnancy in women taking valproate).

Potential parents are also often concerned about the risk of their children themselves developing epilepsy. A precisely quantified risk is usually impossible, but a broad overview figure is 8 per cent if only the mother is affected, 4 per cent if only the father is affected and 25 per cent if both parents have epilepsy (*see* Chapter 5).

During pregnancy

For patients not already under specialist care, **the first antenatal visit** provides an opportunity to set the right therapeutic path for the pregnancy. Ideally, an epilepsy specialist nurse liaising closely with the booking midwife will see the woman at this point and provide the necessary information, support and telephone contact.

Anti-epileptic medication, if considered necessary, should be continued as for the preconception regimen.

Folate 5 mg daily should be continued until after the first trimester.

Screening for neural tube defects by blood and ultrasound testing is appropriate for all women taking anti-epileptic medication, particularly valproate or carbamazepine.

Anti-epileptic **blood level measurement** is often considered in pregnancy, especially for patients taking carbamazepine or phenytoin. The total serum level of anti-epileptic medications falls in pregnancy, especially during the first and third trimesters. This is due to an increased plasma volume, a reduced plasma albumin level and increased hepatic and renal clearance. The potential fall in free drug levels is, however, counterbalanced by reduced protein binding increasing the level of free drug. Thus, a change in total (protein-bound) serum concentration is not itself an indication to change the prescribed dose.

The role of routine repeated serum level testing in pregnancy, as sometimes advised, is unclear. It is probably better to continue to make medication decisions during pregnancy on clinical grounds unless there is evidence of possible toxicity or poor compliance.

Vitamin K supplementation, 20 mg orally daily, is necessary in the last month of pregnancy for women taking liver enzyme-inducing medications, such as carbamazepine or phenytoin. Vitamin K injection is also advised for the newborn. These measures are aimed at preventing bleeding abnormalities in the newborn. Vitamin K throughout pregnancy has been suggested for women taking phenytoin (Howe *et al.*, 1995) in an effort to prevent associated facial anomalies.

Management of labour

- **Delivery method.** A normal vaginal delivery is appropriate for the large majority of cases. Elective caesarean section may have to be considered in patients with frequent tonic-clonic seizures in pregnancy.
- **Seizures** during labour occur in about 1–2 per cent of women with epilepsy. Most do not require specific treatment. If serial seizures occur, lorazepam is the treatment of choice. Intravenous phenytoin, normally a first-line treatment for status epilepticus, may, in theory, prolong labour by inhibiting myometrial contraction and must therefore be used with caution.
- **Eclampsia** is no more likely in epilepsy than in other circumstances. The management of eclampsia is described in Chapter 6. Magnesium sulphate is the preferred treatment. For non-eclamptic seizures, however, magnesium is a poor anticonvulsant and, being an inhibitor of uterine activity, may adversely affect the baby.

PARENTHOOD

Minimize the risk to the baby. New mothers must be aware of the possible risk to the newborn child of injury that might result from parental seizures. If the seizures are frequent, nursing, feeding, changing and bathing the child should, as far as possible, be conducted while sitting on the floor surrounded by cushions. Carrying the baby, for example on the stairs, may be best done with the baby strapped into a carrycot.

Minimize sleep loss. The care of a newborn baby inevitably involves disrupted sleep, which may provoke seizures, especially in idiopathic epilepsy.

Breast feeding is still best even for the mother taking anti-epileptic medication. The breast milk concentration of anti-epileptic medications varies with their lipophilic properties and plasma concentrations. The milk:plasma ratio for individual drugs is valproate 0.05, phenytoin 0.10, phenobarbitone 0.40, carbamazepine 0.45 and oxcarbazepine 0.5. Although the drugs do appear in the breast milk, problems are rarely encountered. The baby will still receive considerably less drug from breast milk than he or she received *in utero*.

An accumulation of phenobarbitone (neonatal half-life 40–300 hours) may provoke drowsiness or subsequent withdrawal effects, and if the mother is started on anti-epileptic medication post partum, allergic rashes occasionally occur in the newborn.

INFORMATION FOR PATIENTS

It is essential that women of child-bearing potential are aware of the problems relating to their medication, contraception and pregnancy. Figure 8.1 gives an example of an information sheet that might be used in an epilepsy clinic.

COSMETIC EFFECTS OF ANTI-EPILEPTIC MEDICATION

Although cosmetic effects occur equally in both sexes, women more often voice such concerns than men. Hirsutism and gum hypertrophy are well-recognized side effects of phenytoin (unrelated to the dose or duration of treatment), as are chloasma, acne and subcutaneous tissue changes (e.g. coarsened features with thickening of the facial skin). Phenytoin is therefore best avoided in women, particularly adolescent girls. Valproate, especially in a high dose, may cause weight gain so must be prescribed with caution in overweight or weight-conscious individuals.

BONE HEALTH

Any drug taken by women or children that alters bone mineral metabolism may compromise bone health. The established anti-epileptic medications are

Figure 8.1
Information sheet for young women with epilepsy

Most pregnancies in women with epilepsy are entirely uneventful and result in healthy children. Below are some answers to frequently asked questions. We would be happy to discuss these with you further in the clinic.

Is the contraceptive pill safe to use with anti-epileptic medication?
If you take carbamazepine, oxcarbazepine, phenytoin or topiramate, you will need a higher oestrogen dosed pill (50 micrograms instead of the usual 30 micrograms). You should consider additional methods of contraception when taking these medications.

Do seizures during pregnancy harm the unborn baby?
This risk is not known. Minor seizures ought not to be harmful. Major seizures may possibly harm the unborn child, either through direct injury or through oxygen shortage during the seizure.

Does epilepsy medication during pregnancy harm the unborn baby?
All anti-epileptic medications are potentially harmful to the unborn child. More is known about the risks of the older medications (e.g. sodium valproate, carbamazepine and phenytoin) and less about the newer treatments (e.g. gabapentin, lamotrigine, levetiracetam, oxcarbazepine, tiagabine, topiramate and vigabatrin); the newer drugs are not necessarily safer.

Significant problems occur in 7–10% of pregnancies on anti-epileptic medication compared with about 5% of pregnancies in which no medication is taken. The risk is highest with larger doses and multiple medications. Most problems arise in early pregnancy, before women even realize they are pregnant.

- **Sodium valproate** (e.g. Epilim) is associated with an increased risk of spina bifida (incomplete development of the spinal cord) in the unborn child. The risk is about 1–2 per 100 births compared with 1 per 1000 if not on medication. The 'fetal valproate syndrome' (minor facial features and slowed development) is rare.
- **Carbamazepine** (e.g. Tegretol) is also associated with an increased risk of spina bifida (1 per 100 births compared with 1 per 1000 if not on medication).
- **Phenytoin** (Epanutin). Uncommon but major problems are heart defects and cleft palate.
- **Newer drugs.** There is insufficient information available to comment adequately on the newer drugs such as gabapentin, lamotrigine, levetiracetam, oxcarbazepine, tiagabine, topiramate and vigabatrin.

Should I take folic acid supplements?
Anti-epileptic drugs can interfere with folate (a B vitamin), and this may contribute to the risk of problems in the baby. Folate supplements can reduce the risk of spina bifida but must be taken before and during early pregnancy.

All women of child-bearing potential taking anti-epileptic medication should also take folic acid 5 mg daily. This needs to be prescribed by your doctor.

Should I take vitamin K supplements?
Vitamin K deficiency causes bleeding in the newborn baby. It may result from taking carbamazepine, phenobarbitone, phenytoin or topiramate in pregnancy.

Women on these medications should take vitamin K 10 mg tablets daily for the final month of pregnancy; their babies should receive a vitamin K injection at birth.

Should I continue taking epilepsy medication during pregnancy?
In a few cases, it is safe to withdraw medication under medical supervision. For most people, treatment must be continued throughout pregnancy.

Please do not stop your medication without first consulting your doctor.

Is it safe to breast feed while taking anti-epileptic medication?
The baby will have already received some medication in the womb. The small amount in the breast milk is not considered harmful.

Breast feeding is advised for all women, including those with epilepsy.

What precautions are needed in caring for a newborn baby?
If seizures are frequent, consider:

- Feeding and changing the baby on the floor surrounded by cushions.
- Bathing the baby in very shallow water with the bath on the floor.
- Using a carrycot to strap in and carry the baby, particularly on stairs.
- Not lying on the bed holding your baby.
- Getting enough rest and sleep; disturbed sleep can trigger seizures.

What is the chance of my child developing epilepsy?
The risk is small and cannot be predicted exactly for any couple. The overall risk is:

- Up to 1 per cent if neither parent has epilepsy.
- Up to 8 per cent if the mother has epilepsy.
- Up to 4 per cent if the father has epilepsy.
- Up to 25 per cent if both parents have epilepsy.

Where can I find further information?

- British Epilepsy Association, Tel: 0800 309030

**If you have further questions or would like more information,
PLEASE ASK.**

associated with an increased risk of osteoporosis, osteomalacia and fractures. The traditional view is that this results predominantly from inducing the metabolism of vitamin D to inactive metabolites; this does not, however, explain why valproate, not an enzyme inducer, should also affect bone density (Sheth *et al.*, 1995). Interference with calcium absorption and an altered cellular responsiveness to parathormone have been postulated.

Anti-epileptic medication alone is rarely responsible for significant osteomalacia and osteoporosis, but, in combination with other risk factors, these problems may occur.

Epilepsy and the elderly

Many people are surprised to learn that epilepsy is more common in the elderly than at any other age, being the third most common neurological disorder in old age after dementia and stroke (Tallis, 1995). One per cent of the over-60s have epilepsy, and evidence suggests that this proportion is increasing (Sander *et al.*, 1990). With a rapidly expanding elderly population (20 per cent of the world population will be over 65 years by 2050 [Scheure, 1995]), epilepsy represents a major and increasing clinical and public health problem.

Furthermore, epilepsy in the elderly is potentially more serious than in younger age groups, for several reasons:

- The **risk of injury** from falls during a seizure is increased owing to frailty, including osteoporotic fractures.
- **Difficulty in diagnosis** owing to co-morbidity may lead to a delay in the recognition of epilepsy.
- **Age-related pharmacokinetic changes** (slowed metabolism and excretion) require a reduced daily dose of medication in the elderly.
- **Side effects** from medication are more common, often because of the slowed metabolism and excretion; the long-term bone health consequences of enzyme-inducing drugs such as phenytoin or carbamazepine are a particular problem in the elderly.
- **Polypharmacy** is common, increasing the risk of anti-epileptic drug interactions.
- **Post-ictal confusion** is often more prolonged in the elderly.
- **Mortality** from convulsive status epilepticus is high (over 30 per cent) in the elderly.
- The **confidence** of an elderly person may be seriously damaged by epilepsy, severely limiting his or her physical activity and social contact.

SEIZURE TYPES

Acute symptomatic (provoked) seizures are more common in the elderly than in the general adult population. Metabolic and toxic causes account for about 10 per cent of seizures in the over-65 years age group. Common epileptogenic factors include medication toxicity (especially from antidepressants or antipsychotic drugs), medication withdrawal (especially of benzodiazepines), alcohol toxicity or withdrawal, metabolic causes, head injury, hypotension, infection and subdural haematoma.

EPILEPSY TYPES

The majority of seizures occurring for the first time in the elderly are of clinically partial onset, with or without secondary generalization. It follows that almost all newly diagnosed cases of epilepsy in the elderly will, where classification is possible, be designated as symptomatic or cryptogenic localization-related epilepsy, with very few 'idiopathic' types.

AETIOLOGY

The increased incidence of seizures in the elderly reflects the increased prevalence of underlying structural brain lesions; there is also some evidence to suggest an increased susceptibility of the ageing brain to seizures. Four causes are most commonly identified:

- **Cerebrovascular disease.** This is the most commonly imputed cause for elderly-onset epilepsy, being responsible for 75 per cent of cases in which a definite cause is identified (Sander *et al.*, 1990). White matter lesions on brain imaging are common but usually represent an incidental finding in elderly persons, although they perhaps serve as a marker for inapparent epileptogenic cortical vascular lesions.
- **Brain tumours.** Tumours underlie 10–15 per cent of elderly-onset epilepsy, mostly metastases or inoperable gliomas with a poor overall prognosis (Lundorf *et al.*, 1986).
- **Dementia.** Seizures may be an early or even a presenting feature of progressive dementia (McAreavey *et al.*, 1992).
- **Head injury.** As in any age group, the late effects of previous head injury may lead to epilepsy, often proving resistant to medication.

PROBLEMS IN DIAGNOSING EPILEPSY

As in any patient group, the diagnosis of blackouts is clinical and centred upon the history. A witness history from family members or carers is particularly important. Several practical difficulties in diagnosing blackouts are apparent in this population.

- An **inadequate history** may be all that is available. The history of blackouts given by an elderly person living alone is often incomplete and lacking a witness account. A history of trauma may be inapparent, even in patients shown to have a subdural haematoma.
- **Falls** are common in the elderly; a seizure as the cause may not be considered.
- **Co-morbidity** is common (cardiac and other cerebral diseases), making the cause of the blackouts uncertain.
- **Polypharmacy** is common and occasionally is the cause of blackouts.
- **Non-convulsive status**, more common in the elderly than in other adult age groups, may present as intermittent confusion without obvious seizure manifestations.

DIFFERENTIAL DIAGNOSIS OF BLACKOUTS

The differential diagnosis of paroxysmal events in the elderly is often unclear at the outset. Diagnostic uncertainty commonly persists in the elderly patient despite a detailed investigation. The main confusion arises between seizures and cardiovascular events.

Drop attacks

Falls are common in the elderly, the majority being due to accidental or environmental factors as well as weakness, ataxia or gait disorder. Drop attacks are falls in which the cause is uncertain, the event unexpected and consciousness is retained (Dey and Kenny, 1997). Drop attacks in the elderly are predominantly cardiovascular, usually caused by age-related autonomic dysfunction leading to orthostatic hypotension. Detailed cardiovascular investigation, including tilt table testing and carotid sinus massage, may be necessary to reach the diagnosis.

Syncope

Syncope is particularly likely to lead to diagnostic confusion. Postural hypotension (often age related and exacerbated by medication), micturition syncope, carotid sinus syncope, arrhythmia and heart block are relatively common in the elderly. Tonic stiffening, jerks, incontinence and injury may all accompany syncope. The atheromatous narrowing of a major vessel might even produce focal symptoms or signs, for example focal jerking, during a hypotensive episode. The common finding of ischaemic heart disease or an abnormality of atrioventricular conduction can lead to diagnostic confusion.

Sleep disorders

Sleep disorders such as obstructive sleep apnoea may cause daytime somnolence and sometimes confusion owing to sleep deprivation. Such patients, unlike those with seizures, can quickly be roused to normal. Narcolepsy and cataplexy may sometimes be diagnosed for the first time in the elderly. Nocturnal confusion is a common early feature of dementia and must be distinguished from complex partial seizures. REM sleep behaviour disorder is a rare condition usually seen in elderly patients, especially those with brainstem pathology: dreams are acted out, sometimes with violent and apparently confused behaviour in sleep.

Transient ischaemic attacks

Transient ischaemic attacks (TIAs) are commonly misdiagnosed as seizures in the elderly, and vice versa. Altered consciousness is rare in a TIA, occurring only in brainstem ischaemia, when other brainstem symptoms (vertigo, vomiting and ataxia) are to be expected. TIA symptoms are usually negative (numbness or weakness) compared with the positive symptoms of epilepsy (jerking and automatism). When sensory or motor symptoms occur in seizures, they are generally briefer and more localized than in TIAs.

Other differential diagnoses

- **Tremor** in the elderly may occasionally be sufficiently prominent to suggest a continued focal seizure.
- **Confusional states** are common in the elderly; non-convulsive status is easily overlooked.
- **Migraine aura** without headache (migraine equivalent) rarely presents for the first time in the elderly.
- **Psychogenic non-epileptic attack disorder** is rare in old age and must be diagnosed in this group only with great caution.

STATUS EPILEPTICUS

- **Tonic-clonic status epilepticus** is serious and often resistant to treatment in the elderly, the higher mortality in this group also reflecting the underlying cause.
- **Complex partial status epilepticus** is an important treatable cause of confusion in the elderly; a suspicion of this condition is a clear indication for recording an EEG.

INVESTIGATIONS

Physical examination in elderly patients with undiagnosed blackouts should include a neurological examination and a detailed assessment of cardiovascular function, including lying and standing blood pressure and pulse rate measurement.

In terms of **investigations**, consideration should be given to a measurement of blood sugar, other electrolytes and erythrocyte sedimentation rate, and to an ECG. In principle, all elderly patients presenting with unprovoked seizures should undergo a brain scan, preferably MRI. An EEG can often help in localizing the seizure focus. Unfortunately, brain scan and EEG results are often equivocal since minor, often incidental, abnormalities are common and their relevance difficult to determine.

MANAGEMENT

Diagnosis

Certainty of diagnosis is essential – all the more so in this age group because the potential for side effects from anti-epileptic medication is greater than in the younger population. The treatment of underlying medical problems or stopping epileptogenic medication (e.g. tricyclic antidepressants) is sometimes sufficient to prevent seizure recurrence.

Lack of trial evidence

Despite the large number of elderly patients with epilepsy, there are very few controlled clinical trials of epilepsy management in this age group; elderly patients are usually excluded from trials of new anti-epileptic medications, limiting the choice of validated anti-epileptic medication. Nevertheless, the same principles of anti-epileptic treatment apply to the elderly as to any other age group.

Whom to treat?

The decision to treat spontaneous seizures in the elderly must take account of their higher chance of seizure recurrence and their risk of injury. This must be balanced against their greater vulnerability to drug interactions and side effects, and the risk of poor compliance. Acute symptomatic seizures will require anti-epileptic treatment only in the short term, if at all. Status epilepticus is, as at any age, a medical emergency, with a significantly increased mortality in the elderly, and requires aggressive intervention.

Which medication?

A reasonable choice of medication for the elderly would be sodium valproate or lamotrigine, since both have a broad spectrum of anti-epileptic action, few sedative side effects, few interactions except with other anti-epileptic drugs, and no effect on bone health. Gabapentin shares several of these advantages, although it is only for partial-onset seizures. Oxcarbazepine is preferred to carbamazepine in the elderly owing to its lesser tendency towards producing sedative side effects and rash, but caution is still needed regarding the possibility of hyponatraemia.

Dosing regimen

If long-term medication is necessary, a low dose of monotherapy prescribed in no more than a twice daily dosing regimen is appropriate for most patients. The appropriate dose is, in general, decided on clinical grounds; blood levels are rarely needed unless using phenytoin or if unexpected side effects are suspected with other medications.

There are several reasons for caution in prescribing anti-epileptic medications to the elderly.

- **Carbamazepine** side effects, including its potential for interactions, hyponatraemia and the exacerbation of atrioventricular conduction block, may be more likely in the elderly.
- **Valproate** daily dosage should be reduced in this group owing to its reduced excretion rate.
- **Phenytoin** had long been the preferred choice because of its low cost, once daily dosing and prompt action when given parenterally in an acute situation. It is, however, difficult to use owing to its saturation kinetics and age-related changes in metabolism. Blood levels are therefore needed to optimize the dose, but even these are only ever a guide and can be misleading, particularly in the elderly. Even when a satisfactory level is established, it is easily upset by interaction with additional medications or by intercurrent illness, both common at this age.
- **Phenobarbitone** is not recommended as, in the elderly, it is particularly likely to lead to oversedation or paradoxical central nervous system excitation.
- **Enzyme-inducing drugs** such as phenytoin and phenobarbitone may also worsen a pre-existing propensity to osteoporosis and osteomalacia.

PROGNOSIS

Despite the prevalence of epilepsy in the elderly, there are relatively few data on prognosis, the effect of treatment and the success of medication withdrawal in this population. Overall, however, the prognosis for epilepsy and mortality is worse in the elderly than in younger populations. The risk of seizure recurrence at 1 year following a single seizure in patients over the age of 60 years is 80 per cent compared with 70 per cent in the remaining adult population (Hart *et al.*, 1990). The considerably greater mortality in elderly compared to younger patients with epilepsy is because of the different seizure aetiology, for example underlying metastatic tumour or stroke.

Special issues in epilepsy

Psychosocial aspects

Psychosocial problems are associated with any chronic illness, but there are special considerations when that illness is epilepsy. Indeed, the medical aspects of epilepsy are not necessarily the most important to the patient. The problems of epilepsy can be divided into impairment (the disease), disability (the illness) and handicap (the predicaments) (Taylor, 1996).

The **impairment** (disease) is the organ, i.e. the brain, problem. There are specific changes in the structural or functional organization of tissue, and scope for specific therapy and for reconciliation to the condition. The impairment of epilepsy is the tendency to develop seizures.

The **disability** (illness) is the 'whole person' problem. It is the declaration of disease, characterized by a social manifestation, a role which can be modified by developmental processes and in which there is scope for palliation and for personal change. The disability of epilepsy is the inability to perform physically and mentally because of the seizure tendency.

The **handicap** (predicament) is the 'socio-economic' problem, the complex of psychosocial ramifications with immediate bearing on the individual. These are diffuse, multifactorial and personal but not necessarily unique. There is scope for social and political remedies for predicaments, which can be major in someone with epilepsy. The handicap of epilepsy is the restricted opportunity for personal development, reduced confidence and self-esteem, and generally a lower quality of life.

It is too easy to concentrate on the disease while ignoring the illness and predicaments. The degree of handicap is influenced by social, physical, economic and personal factors. The loss of a driving licence, for example, is a vastly greater handicap to people living in an isolated rural environment than to those in an urban area with easy access to public transport. Lack of social contact is a major source of dissatisfaction. Patients may feel too frightened to go out, or their anxieties may interfere with their social performance. The reaction of their family may also add to their handicap if parents are anxious and overprotective and impose inappropriate restrictions.

FAMILY REACTION TO CHILDHOOD EPILEPSY

The stresses to which the family is subjected as a result of a child's epilepsy can only be individualized if there is a good understanding of the way in which the chronically sick child is received within the family, the family's perception of the child and its handling of the situation. For all children, full pregnancy, birth, developmental, medical and family histories are as essential for psychiatric assessment as for the management of the disease.

- **Carer role.** The major implications of parenting a chronically sick child require attention.
- **Grief.** The parents will feel the loss of a perfect child.
- **Fear.** Epileptic seizures are very frightening occurrences: most parents, at the first generalized tonic-clonic seizure, and often at subsequent ones, think that their children are dying.
- **Guilt.** This is a common factor, particularly in conditions that are chronic, related to the nervous system and possibly of genetic significance.
- **Concern about learning disability.** The association of epilepsy with learning difficulties is well recognized among lay people, many believing that a diagnosis of epilepsy automatically implies that there will be educational difficulties.
- **Denial.** There is often a denial or repression of the possibility of a brain disorder.
- **Reaction formation**, with an extreme degree of commitment to the affected child and a lack of appreciation of the needs of the self or others in the family, can occur.
- **Displacement**, or the diversion of distress from the child to professionals, leads to recurring disappointment as the return of the perfect child is never achieved.

RESTRICTIONS

The wider experiences of children with epilepsy are likely to be curtailed:

- **Risk taking.** Children are discouraged from taking risks, including swimming and cycling.
- **Exploration.** They do not have opportunities for independent exploration and thus lack environmental information that would normally be acquired.
- **Friendships.** These are more difficult to make.
- **Independence.** The level of supervision usually accorded to a child with seizures, together with the increased risk of seizures (even if, in many cases, this risk is minimal), restricts their independence and renders them more vulnerable.
- **Social skills.** Social skills suffer as a result.

SOCIAL PROBLEMS

Several factors contribute to the social problems of people with epilepsy.

People with epilepsy consistently fail to realize their **educational potential**, for two main reasons:

- **Medical:** drug side effects, recurrent seizures and organic impairments of memory or language;
- **Social:** lowered expectations, overprotection, time off school and missed opportunities.

The **unemployment** rate is invariably higher in economically active patients with epilepsy (50 per cent) compared with age-matched and sex-matched controls (20 per cent). Employment opportunities are limited according to seizure type, seizure frequency, educational background and employer attitude.

Driving is forbidden to people with an active liability to seizures, adding considerably to their social disadvantage.

The **overprotection** of children with epilepsy leads to their greater dependency and a slower development of personality and social skills than occurs in the general population.

Negative **stigmatizing attitudes** of society towards epilepsy – both actual and perceived – lead to a general inability to fulfil a person's potential. The result may be poorer interpersonal skills, greater social isolation, less involvement in leisure activities and a lower rate of marriage.

Anxiety, **depression**, personality disorder and even psychosis may lead to social disadvantage and exclusion.

The stigma of epilepsy

Stigma exists when an individual is perceived as being unacceptably different from the 'normal' people with whom he or she routinely interacts, and with this goes some form of community sanction. Disease-related stigma varies at different times and between cultures. In the twentieth century, for example, cancer replaced tuberculosis as the most feared and stigmatized disorder. Diseases that are visible and intrusive, and particularly those considered to be mental disorders, are the most stigmatizing. Patients with epilepsy are therefore vulnerable to considerable stigma.

Many patients with epilepsy sense a stigma ('felt stigma') well before experiencing any actual hostile reaction from others ('enacted stigma'). Seizures are often too infrequent (particularly outside the home) to give many opportunities for enacted stigma. It is thus more often the perception of stigma than the actual reaction of others that is the main disruption to the life of a person with epilepsy (Scambler, 1998).

The surest way to end stigma is to find the causes and to treat the illness effectively. The enormous strides in the understanding of the causes of epilepsy and the wealth of new treatments (including surgery) offer real hope for today's patients diagnosed with epilepsy. Newer drugs offer treatment that is far less stigmatizing (particularly because of fewer cosmetic and sedative side effects) than that encountered in previous generations. With each advance, we can hope for a more enlightened attitude to the many and varied disorders collectively known as epilepsy.

Driving

The loss of a driving licence often contributes most to the handicap of epilepsy. Driving restriction is a major source of patient dissatisfaction with a consultation for epilepsy. In most aspects of living with epilepsy (employment, sport and leisure), the restrictions are voluntary and negotiable. With driving, however, clear restrictive legislation must be followed.

ORDINARY LICENCE

The current UK driving regulations for people with epilepsy are as follows.

One-year rule
Following an unprovoked epileptic seizure (or an undiagnosed blackout), a driver should be advised to stop driving immediately and to inform the DVLA of the event. There must be freedom from seizures for 1 year before the licence is restored. Patients must also be considered not to be a danger to the public, i.e. honest in their declaration of the date of their last seizure and without other factors (e.g. drug-related sedative side effects) that might interfere with their driving ability. Knowingly failing to advise the DVLA is an offence and effectively invalidates the driving licence and vehicle insurance for that driver.

Three-year rule
A special rule for patients who have only sleep-related seizures is that, although following initial attacks they must stop driving until they are seizure free for 1 year, they may resume driving despite continued seizures provided that they have an established pattern of sleep-related seizures for 3 years.

VOCATIONAL LICENCE

This applies to drivers of heavy goods vehicles (HGV = greater than 7.5 tonnes laden weight) and public service vehicles (PSV = more than nine seats for hire or reward), as well as to taxi drivers.

To hold such a licence, drivers must fulfil all of the following criteria:

- 10 years or more of freedom from seizures;
- 10 years or more off all anti-epileptic medication;
- not considered to be a danger to the public.

The following points apply to driving and epilepsy in the UK.

The onus for informing the DVLA lies with the driver

The doctor's role is to advise the patient to comply with the regulations and therefore to stop driving and inform the DVLA. It is not the doctor who imposes the driving ban but the DVLA, upon receiving information from the patient. Drivers must be aware that both driving licence and insurance are invalid should they continue driving. In a minority of cases, the doctor may inform the DVLA without the patient's consent. Such a breach of medical confidence may be justified by a greater duty to the community, and in doing so the doctor would be supported by the General Medical Council. Doctors must clearly document in the notes the advice given to patients about driving.

Single seizure

Although not epilepsy, a single unprovoked seizure carries a sufficient risk of recurrent seizures to justify the same duration of driving ban as if it were epilepsy.

Provoked seizures

Seizures provoked by other medical conditions, for example eclampsia, and by anaesthesia, are dealt with (usually leniently) on an individual basis by the DVLA; the full epilepsy regulations are not necessarily applied.

Alcohol and illicit drug-related seizures

Although these are provoked, they nevertheless usually result in a 1-year driving ban.

Syncope

Patients rarely faint while driving and, for the large majority of patients, simple syncope does not need to be reported to the DVLA. Brief myoclonia frequently accompanies a faint (Lempert *et al.*, 1994); this does not necessarily imply a post-anoxic seizure, nor does it need to be reported. DVLA advice should, however, be sought for patients whose faints are atypical, who habitually faint with little warning or from the recumbent posture, or who have a definite seizure following a severe syncopal episode.

Medication

For an ordinary driving licence, it does not matter whether patients are on or off medication: it is the date of the last seizure that counts.

Reflex epilepsy

Some epilepsies, for example photosensitive epilepsy and reading epilepsy, are provoked only in certain situations; patients with these epilepsies must nevertheless meet the epilepsy regulations.

Seizures with retained consciousness

The present UK driving regulations do not distinguish between seizures with or without a loss of consciousness. Auras and myoclonic jerks count as seizures in the eyes of the DVLA. A licence holder must report any seizure event and be seizure free for 1 year before resuming driving.

Tumours

The duration of the driving ban increases to between 1 and 4 years depending upon the degree of malignancy of the tumour.

Head injury

Seizures occurring immediately following an acute head injury (immediate 'concussive' seizures) do not predict later epilepsy so the DVLA will usually allow driving to resume. Seizures occurring at any time other than immediately after the injury are associated with a significantly increased risk of subsequent epilepsy, so the epilepsy driving regulations apply.

Craniotomy

Patients who have undergone craniotomy involving a penetration of the dura are deemed to be at sufficient risk of epileptic seizures to be advised to stop driving and inform the DVLA, whether or not they have ever had an epileptic seizure.

Visual fields and epilepsy

Certain situations in epilepsy may sufficiently impair the field of vision to preclude driving even if the epilepsy regulations are met. The current regulations insist upon 120 degrees of binocular horizontal vision and 20 degrees above and below the horizontal before driving is permitted. Patients previously treated with vigabatrin may have significant and permanent visual field restriction. In addition, patients who have previously undergone temporal lobectomy for seizure control are commonly left with an homonymous upper quadrantanopia. Both situations might preclude legally holding a driving licence.

The EEG

This is a surprisingly poor predictor of future seizures and has almost no role in deciding an individual's driving restriction. In the special case of typical absence epilepsy (rare in adults), the finding of three-per-second spike-and-wave activity on the EEG is sufficient to impose a 1-year driving ban.

Common excuses

Drivers commonly state that they drive only short distances, that they have adequate warning of an attack, that they have never had an attack when driving or that they had a seizure only because they had forgotten to take a tablet or had received an incorrect prescription. None of these explanations is likely to prevent the DVLA from imposing the standard epilepsy regulations.

Medication withdrawal

If anti-epileptic medication is being withdrawn from a driver who is seizure free, the DVLA advises, although does not insist, that driving ceases from the time of starting drug withdrawal until 6 months after the cessation of treatment.

DO PATIENTS INFORM THE DRIVING AUTHORITIES?

Many ineligible people continue to drive despite advice to the contrary from their clinician. A recent study found that about 70 per cent of patients with epilepsy failed to inform the DVLA as advised (Taylor *et al.*, 1995). The present system of self-reporting is therefore not particularly effective.

DOES EPILEPSY CAUSE ROAD ACCIDENTS AND DEATH?

Perhaps surprisingly, the overall accident rate is no different in eligible drivers with or without a history of epilepsy. The big difference is that, should they have an accident, drivers with epilepsy are at a 40 per cent increased risk of causing a serious injury or fatality. Patients often protest that the law is unfair because they have a warning of their seizures so could take evasive action should a fit begin. The risk of accident, however, appears to be independent of a history of aura, and independent of whether patients are taking anti-epileptic medication, and of whether or not there has been a fit in the past 3 years.

Employment

The adult with poorly controlled seizures is at a considerable disadvantage in the job market. High levels of unemployment and underemployment exist among people with epilepsy. Unemployment has more than just economic implications: employment gives a structure to people's lives, feelings of self-worth and an identity within society.

OFFICIAL BARRIERS TO EMPLOYMENT

Certain occupations are inaccessible to patients with epilepsy. The restrictions vary between countries and may vary even in one line of employment within a country. Career restrictions may be divided into absolute, relative and individual:

- **Absolute.** People in the UK wishing to become an aircraft pilot or to join the air force (with few exceptions), the navy or the fire service must have had no established medical history or clinical diagnosis of epilepsy at any time in their lives.
- **Relative.** People in the UK seeking employment involving heavy goods vehicle, public service vehicle or taxi driving must fulfil the appropriate regulations so must have been seizure free and off medication for 10 years. People entering the ambulance service or army, or wishing to become a diver, merchant seaman or train driver (regulations differ among different rail companies), must normally have had no seizures since the age of 5 years.
- **Individual.** Patients wishing to become a nurse, midwife or teacher, or to join the police, prison or coast guard service, are assessed individually. These professions often take the ordinary driving licence rules – 1 year seizure free on or off treatment – as their guide.

UNOFFICIAL BARRIERS TO EMPLOYMENT

The greatest obstacles faced by people with epilepsy seeking employment are unofficial and often unspoken. Discrimination in the workplace against persons with epilepsy persists, mainly through misinformation and misconception.

First is **employer misconception**. Popular perceptions of epilepsy are often incorrect. Epilepsy is too often perceived as a single, unchanging and usually convulsive entity. Lay opinion is formed from a limited knowledge of one extreme of the epilepsy spectrum, i.e. major convulsions with risk of injury in severely handicapped people. Thus, employers, like many members of the public, are fearful and even hostile towards people with epilepsy. They may have particular, but usually unfounded, fears that seizures might be provoked by their work, for example by using VDUs, or that people with epilepsy have a high sickness rate. They may have disproportionate concerns about self-injury during a seizure, although safety regulations should ensure that machines are adequately guarded for all workers whether or not they have epilepsy.

There are also **employee misconceptions**. People with epilepsy often feel that their job prospects are very limited. Negative expectations at interview may influence their presentation: a self-fulfilling prophecy.

SHOULD PATIENTS DISCLOSE THEIR EPILEPSY TO EMPLOYERS?

Many people correctly believe that the disclosure of epilepsy harms their prospects in securing employment. Failure to disclose epilepsy, however, is a legitimate reason for dismissal if the epilepsy is a specific impediment to a particular type of work. The concealment of a major medical problem is rarely helpful, and the anxiety resulting from non-disclosure may itself impair quality of life and reinforce the fear of stigmatization.

On balance, patients are best advised to inform their employers but need advice in choosing the right way and the right time to do so; leaving a blank on the application form with the intention of discussing the seizure history at interview is one possibility.

School

The range of cognitive abilities in children with epilepsy is as wide as it is in the general population. For almost all, the appropriate school will be identified on the basis of educational potential rather than on factors related to the epilepsy. Nevertheless, the child with frequent seizures could require medical attention during school hours, and this may need to be acknowledged in choosing the school placement. In addition, for those with physical disabilities such as cerebral palsy, education might be better delivered in a school that permits easy access for those with walking aids or wheelchairs. Thus, as for all other special issues in epilepsy, the seizures are but one facet that needs to be considered.

STATEMENT OF EDUCATIONAL NEEDS

Attempts are currently made to educate all children in mainstream schools with individualized support. However, many children with learning and other disabilities continue to attend special establishments that are considered to be more suited to their needs than mainstream schools.

Educational psychologists, teachers, community paediatricians and parents identify the type of educational support required. Physiotherapists, occupational therapists, speech therapists, paediatric neurologists, etc., may provide further information. The result is a Statement of Educational Needs. Once a child has a Statement, this must, by law, be reviewed annually so that changes in need are identified on a regular basis. The Statement will recommend the type of school considered to be appropriate, often naming a specific school, and, for children who remain in mainstream classes, the extra help that they should receive there.

OPTIONS FOR SCHOOLING

State (non-fee-paying) schools
The school types within the state system are as follows:

- mainstream;
- mainstream with a special unit: these may cater for pupils with learning difficulties, but are often more for those with specific sensory difficulties, such as visual or hearing deficits;
- schools for children with moderate learning difficulties;
- schools for children with severe learning disabilities;
- schools with special facilities for the physically handicapped (which usually also have many pupils with moderate learning difficulties in addition to handicaps that are predominantly physical);
- establishments for children with severe behavioural difficulties.

Private (fee-paying) schools
Most fee-paying schools have difficulty in catering for children with learning or other specific problems, although a small number are able to provide appropriate facilities.

Residential special schools
In the UK, there is a small number of residential schools where there is special expertise in the understanding and management of epilepsy and its educational implications. Only 0.5 per cent of children with epilepsy are educated in these schools, but some of them also provide short-term (about 16- week) periods of multidisciplinary assessment. This can be very useful in making recommendations regarding the education services near the child's home.

Special requirements specifically related to epilepsy

Teacher awareness
The parents or carers should ensure that the child's teachers are aware of the epilepsy.

Knowledge of typical attacks

A description of a typical seizure or seizures should be written down and given to a named person in school.

Seizure frequency

The current seizure frequency, giving some estimation of the likelihood of a seizure occurring during school hours, should be available. It is just as important that the school is aware of sleep-related attacks as of those which habitually occur during waking hours: children often fall asleep on the way back from school outings. Weeks away from home, sleeping in hostels while on adventure courses or skiing trips, are also commonplace.

What to do for a seizure

Instructions on what to do if a seizure occurs in school, with a contact telephone number for a parent or a designated substitute, are essential. The usual duration of a seizure is important information.

Diazepam

For those children whose seizures do not terminate spontaneously, rectal diazepam may need to be given, although attempts are being made to assess whether nasal or buccal midazolam would be an adequate alternative. For patients whose need for rectal diazepam can be anticipated, a supply should be kept available in school. In addition, a member of the school staff, usually the school nurse, must be trained in the administration of the diazepam. In rare cases, a teacher will take on this role, after suitable instruction.

Medication effects on cognition

Teachers often attribute learning, concentration and behavioural difficulties to the medication that the child is receiving. The positive benefits of the control of clinical and subclinical seizures may need to be emphasized. Unfounded negative references to drug treatment should be discouraged.

Awareness of cognitive problems

Underachievement in relation to overall ability is common; specific cognitive difficulties should thus be considered and assessed.

Restrictions

The child should be encouraged to participate in all aspects of school life, but special precautions are necessary in relation to apparatus work in physical education and to swimming lessons. For the latter, it should be recognized that the ability to swim is just as important for someone with epilepsy as for anyone else, but that there should always be an adult in the water who has one-to-one responsibility for the child.

In summary, educational placement is usually recommended on the basis of cognitive abilities, but frequent seizures, physical disabilities and behavioural problems may also influence the final decisions about schooling.

Sport and leisure

The spectrum of epilepsy is so broad that generalizations about restrictions for an individual are inappropriate:

- Full and normal participation in sport and leisure should be encouraged in patients with epilepsy.
- The decision to participate lies with the individual rather than the doctor. Too often, patients live an unnecessarily restricted existence upon a doctor's advice.
- Normal living includes living with risks. The risk of having a seizure (which may be high) must be distinguished from the risk of causing injury (which may be quite low). The frequency and type of seizure will clearly influence the advice given. Patients should ask themselves, 'Is this sensible, given my particular condition and level of control?'

INDIVIDUAL ACTIVITIES

Swimming

People with active epilepsy should be encouraged to learn to swim and to do so in properly managed swimming pools. Someone who knows that they have epilepsy and can rescue them if necessary should accompany them. It is usual to advise that an adult (with one-to-one responsibility) always accompanies a child with epilepsy in the water. Common sense must be applied when considering swimming alone, swimming in the sea, rivers or lakes, or sub-aqua diving.

Cycling

For most patients with epilepsy, cycling is enjoyable, sensible and safe. If epilepsy were poorly controlled, however, common sense would dictate the avoidance of riding on busy roads or cycling alone. Everybody, whether or not they have epilepsy, should wear helmets when cycling.

Sports involving isolation

Horse riding, hill walking, mountain biking, sailing, etc. can be undertaken by people with epilepsy, although the level of supervision should reflect the frequency and severity of the seizures. Isolation, for example when hill walking, may clearly present a particular danger should altered consciousness occur.

Contact sports

A common misconception is that head injury is more detrimental to a patient with epilepsy than to one without. There is no reason for this to be the case. Rugby and other contact sports do not need to be avoided in people with epilepsy – what safer place to have a seizure than in the company of 29 other players and a referee? Few doctors, especially neurologists, would advocate boxing, but the decision to box as an amateur should be left with the patient. People with epilepsy are, however, forbidden to box professionally: a person having a complex partial seizure while boxing risks serious injury.

Dangerous sports

Sports involving a significant risk to self or others should a seizure occur (scuba diving, hang gliding, parachuting, etc.) must be discouraged in people with epilepsy. A seizure while rock climbing or scuba diving (unless there are special arrangements) puts colleagues as well as the patient in danger. Special provision can, however, sometimes be made for people with epilepsy to participate in otherwise forbidden activities, for example by tandem parachuting.

Alcohol

ALCOHOL-RELATED SEIZURES

Alcohol may influence epilepsy in several ways:

Toxicity

Alcohol is anti-epileptic but may provoke seizures in susceptible individuals after consuming a large quantity. It is essential to exclude alcohol-induced hypoglycaemia or unrecognized head injury in this situation.

Withdrawal

A common cause of epileptic seizures in people dependent upon a large quantity of alcohol is alcohol withdrawal.

Interference with medications

Alcohol may disrupt the blood level of anti-epileptic medications by interfering with the hepatic metabolism of enzyme-inducing drugs such as carbamazepine, phenytoin and phenobarbitone. One-off alcohol usage may temporarily increase the blood level by competing for metabolic pathways. More importantly, chronic alcohol use will induce liver enzymes and lead to a more rapid metabolism of these medications, thus lowering the blood level and allowing seizures to occur.

Omitting medications

Alcohol is a common cause of missed medications. Patients may vomit or forget to take their tablets if they are intoxicated. Alcohol may provide the spur to an injudicious withdrawal of anti-epileptic medication by increasing the patient's confidence in seizure control. Patients occasionally misinterpret the warning 'not to be taken with alcohol' and deliberately omit their medications if they are planning to drink alcohol.

Impaired sleep quality

Alcohol may interfere with the quality of sleep and thus disrupt seizure control. Although the patient's perception may be of a deep sleep following alcohol, alcohol-induced sleep is characterized by a greatly enhanced tendency for sleep apnoea and frequent arousal, fragmenting sleep and disrupting its quality. Sleep quality is important for epilepsy control, particularly in idiopathic generalized epilepsy such as juvenile myoclonic epilepsy.

Increased seizure morbidity

Alcohol may increase confidence sufficiently to allow patients to be exposed to situations that might potentially provoke seizures and which would otherwise be avoided, for example flashing lights, recreational drugs and late nights. Alcohol may also increase the likelihood of an inappropriate exposure to hazards such as heights and machinery, thereby increasing the risk of serious injury should seizures occur. Alcohol may also increase the probability of aspiration or even death during a seizure.

SAFE DRINKING

Patients with epilepsy should be encouraged to minimize their alcohol consumption. Although abstinence from alcohol is preferred, 2–4 units can be considered to be a safe daily maximum. It is important that patients understand that a larger quantity carries an increased risk of seizures.

Patients taking valproate often recognize that their alcohol tolerance is reduced owing to its tendency for enzyme inhibition.

WHICH MEDICATION TO USE?

Chronic alcohol use will lower the blood levels of liver-metabolized drugs; enzyme-inducing anti-epileptic medications are most likely to interact with alcohol. Sodium valproate is useful in this situation, but, being a potent enzyme inhibitor, it may increase and prolong the sedative effect of alcohol. Alternatives include gabapentin, which is not metabolized in liver.

DRIVING AND ALCOHOL-RELATED SEIZURES

Although alcohol-induced seizures are categorized as 'provoked', the UK driving authority recognizes the high likelihood of recurrence, so takes a very firm line and bans driving for 1 year following such a seizure.

ALCOHOL WITHDRAWAL SEIZURES

Alcohol withdrawal seizures ('rum fits') occur in the context of acute confusion, often with violence, 3–5 days following abrupt alcohol withdrawal, for example following hospital admission for surgery or investigation. These are usually quickly recognized as arising from alcohol withdrawal. Benzodiazepines are usually sufficient to control the acute situation. Thiamine supplements must also be given as Wernicke's encephalopathy can present in a similar way, and the blood sugar level must be checked.

Long-term anti-epileptic medication is not usually required following alcohol withdrawal seizures. Referral for counselling is an important part of the management to try to overcome the problem of alcohol dependence.

Illicit drugs

The recreational use of illicit drugs and other psychoactive substances has become commonplace, particularly among teenagers. Illicit drugs might generally be supposed by doctors and patients adversely to affect seizure threshold and epilepsy, but there are surprisingly few data to support this (Smith and McBride, 1999).

Cocaine

Cocaine appears the most epileptogenic of the available illicit drugs. Large doses (2–5 g), particularly inhaled as 'crack', may cause acute symptomatic seizures even in otherwise healthy people. Young children (e.g. exposed via the passive inhalation of crack cocaine fumes) appear to be at particular risk. The proconvulsant properties of cocaine may be further potentiated by sleep deprivation. Of particular concern is the evidence from animal (Baraban *et al.*, 1997) and retrospective human studies that intrauterine exposure to cocaine increases the risk of subsequent epilepsy in the offspring.

Amphetamines

Amphetamines might in theory be anti-epileptic but in practice lower the seizure threshold through effects on arousal and sleep deprivation. This is particularly important for patients with idiopathic generalized epilepsy, the epilepsy type most prevalent among teenagers. The amphetamine derivative

Ecstasy (3,4-methylenedioxymethamphatamine or MDMA) has become a popular dance drug despite being banned from the UK in 1977. Its use remains widespread despite considerable publicity of altered consciousness, seizures and sometimes death in occasional users. While the seizure risk from Ecstasy comes with its metabolic consequences (especially hyponatraemia), sleep deprivation (as with generic amphetamine) is more often the problem for individuals predisposed to seizures.

Opiates

Opiates such as pethidine, diamorphine and methadone are well known to cause seizures, especially if large doses are received over a short time.

Cannabis

Cannabis, the best known and most widely used of the illicit drugs, has been unconvincingly advocated as an anti-epileptic medication on the basis of occasional single case reports (Consroe *et al.*, 1975). There is, however, no good evidence to suggest that cannabis has either pro-epileptic or anti-epileptic properties, at least in the doses encountered through smoke inhalation. A cannabis user presenting with seizures should therefore be closely questioned about other more likely epileptogenic drugs.

Travel

Advice to patients with epilepsy who travel abroad might include the following:

- Take **adequate tablet supplies** since the names and preparations of tablets obtained abroad might differ from those at home.
- Take **spare tablets** in a separate carrier in case the main supply is lost.
- Carry **accurate written information** about your type of epilepsy and the drugs taken.
- Carry **identification** or a 'Medic Alert' bracelet.
- **Inform the cabin staff** in the aircraft if you are subject to frequent seizures.
- **Alert others** to your epilepsy if you are staying alone when abroad.
- On long haul flights, the change in **time zone** may lead to altered sleep hours and a lack of sleep, which can provoke seizures in susceptible people; also, the tablet regimen can easily become out of step in the new time zone. Try to take the doses of medication within 24-hour periods, much as you would at home. Aim not to leave out any doses.
- All of the commonly used **antimalarial prophylaxis** agents can potentially provoke seizures in susceptible people and so careful thought must be given before prescribing these to people with epilepsy. The risk of malaria and the need for prophylaxis vary considerably between endemic areas and

at different times of year and so specialist advice on individual travel plans is helpful from your travel agent or from the Malaria Prophylaxis Helpline – 020 7636 3924.

Sexuality

Most men and women with epilepsy have a normal and full sexual life, but some problems are encountered in a substantial minority.

HYPOSEXUALITY

Several uncontrolled studies have identified that patients with epilepsy are less sexually active and have a lower libido than patients without epilepsy. This may be especially the case with temporal lobe epilepsy, in those with an onset of seizures in childhood, in those with social maladjustment to their epilepsy and in people with frequent seizures and low intelligence. Enzyme-inducing medication such as carbamazepine and phenytoin may be associated with a change in the level of sexual hormones, including a rise in sex hormone-binding globulin and a fall in androgens in males. The raised level of anxiety in patients with epilepsy, as well as low self-esteem and a (usually unfounded) fear of seizures during intercourse, are also likely to contribute.

SEXUAL SEIZURES

Seizures that manifest as feelings of sexual pleasure or orgasm are rare. They tend to be associated with lesions in the non-dominant hemisphere, in either the paracentral area or the basal temporal area. Symptoms may include a gradual progression to orgasm followed by a loss of consciousness. Sexual activity may also occur during a seizure automatism or during post-ictal confusion.

Crime

The large majority of people with epilepsy are law abiding, the few who are not being driven by the same motives as law breakers who do not have epilepsy. The public perception of crimes committed during epileptic seizures is greatly exaggerated. A very small number of people with epilepsy unwittingly commit crimes during a seizure or in their post-ictal confusion. An example may be picking up something from a shop when confused, or undressing in public. This is normally understood, and no prosecution results. However, if the patient is alone, if there are no other overt manifestations of a seizure, or if aggression and injury occur, then conflict with the law may result.

Mortality

Although epilepsy is rightly considered to be a benign condition, patients with epilepsy have a three times greater risk of death compared with age-matched and sex-matched populations (Cockerell, 1996).

OVERALL MORTALITY

The overall standard mortality ratio of an epilepsy population followed over nearly 7 years was highest in the first year following diagnosis, at 5.1, and declined to 1.3 after 5 years (Cockerell *et al.*, 1994). The mortality rate was much higher for symptomatic compared with cryptogenic epilepsy (4.3 compared with 1.6). This suggests that most of the excess mortality is attributable to serious underlying causes of symptomatic epilepsy, for example cancer and arteriosclerosis, especially in the elderly. Institutionalized patients with epilepsy (often with more severe epilepsy) show almost twice the death rate of epilepsy patients in the community (Nashef *et al.*, 1995).

EPILEPSY-RELATED DEATH

Some deaths are attributable to accidents, suicide or convulsive status epilepticus, but the majority of deaths associated with epilepsy are sudden and unexplained (sudden unexplained death in epilepsy, or SUDEP).

- **Accidental death.** The risk of a fatal accident is higher in the population with epilepsy than in the general population, particularly through drowning while swimming or bathing, but also because of road traffic accidents and other injuries and burns (Spitz *et al.*, 1995). Most such injuries are avoidable.
- **Seizure-related death.** Asphyxiation or aspiration may occur during a seizure.
- **Status epilepticus.** Although rare, this is a serious complication with a mortality of 5–10 per cent, particularly in children and the elderly (*see* Chapter 6).
- **Idiosyncratic reactions.** Reactions to anti-epileptic medications are rare, but fatal cases are occasionally seen, especially in young children.
- **SUDEP** (*see* below).

SUDDEN UNEXPLAINED DEATH IN EPILEPSY

This is an important and not so rare cause of death in patients with epilepsy. It has been known for centuries that people may die during seizures, but only recently has the phenomenon become widely known among doctors and the general public.

Definition
SUDEP is defined as a sudden, unexpected, witnessed or unwitnessed, non-traumatic and non-drowning death in patients with epilepsy, with or without evidence of a seizure and excluding documented status epilepticus, in which post mortem examination does not reveal a toxicological or anatomical cause of death (Nashef, 1997).

Incidence
The incidence of SUDEP is relatively high, lying between 1 in 500 and 1 in 1000 per epilepsy patient per year. Studies of tertiary referral populations give an even higher rate by including more severely affected individuals. In patients awaiting epilepsy surgery, the incidence of SUDEP may be as high as 1 in 100 per year (Dasheiff, 1991). This is itself a major justification for considering epilepsy surgery in patients with medically intractable epilepsy.

Exclusion of known causes
Seizure-related sudden deaths are sometimes explained at autopsy, for example as a blocked airway, a head injury, burns or drowning, but these are not classified as SUDEP. Most SUDEP patients do have evidence of some pulmonary aspiration or pulmonary oedema, but these alone are insufficient to cause death.

Risk factors
Risk factors for SUDEP are suggested by descriptive epidemiology, but definite proof of any specific cause is lacking. Several risk factors for SUDEP (Tennis et al., 1995) are, however, recognized:

- **Age.** Younger patients appear to be most at risk, the mean age at death being 28.6 years (Nashef et al., 1995); the elderly are also probably at risk, but diagnosis is difficult at this age as sudden death is more readily attributed to other causes. The greater susceptibility of young people may reflect an age-related change in cardiorespiratory autonomic reflexes.
- **Sex.** Males are at slightly increased risk compared with females, but some of this difference may reflect social factors, such as excessive alcohol consumption, which could differently influence the mortality rate between the sexes.
- **Seizure type.** Generalized tonic-clonic seizures have occurred in almost all patients succumbing to SUDEP; the implication is that SUDEP itself is associated with generalized tonic-clonic seizures. There is often, but not

invariably, evidence of such a seizure having occurred, for example tongue biting, disrupted bedclothes, etc.

- **Severity of epilepsy.** Patients whose epilepsy is more refractory to treatment, more chronic and more severe are at greater risk of SUDEP. There are exceptions, however, and death has been reported immediately following a first seizure.

- **Compliance.** Poor compliance with medication ought to be an important preventable factor in SUDEP since this would be expected to correlate with poor seizure control. Improving compliance offers some hope of preventing sudden death in high-risk populations. Assessing drug compliance following death is not easy, and there are problems in interpreting a low blood drug level after death owing to a change in body chemistry and cell breakdown. However, the available evidence from post mortem blood anticonvulsant concentrations suggests that poor drug compliance is not a major contributory factor in SUDEP (Opeskin *et al.*, 1999).

- **Neurological deficit and learning disability.** These appear to increase the risk but probably only because of their association with more severe and refractory epilepsy.

- **Seizures in sleep.** About half of SUDEP cases die in their sleep; the reason for this is unknown, but suffocation does not appear to be the answer. It probably relates to the same factors as being alone.

- **Being alone.** Living alone or being unsupervised appears to be a very important risk factor – almost all cases of SUDEP are unwitnessed. The implication is that patients having seizures in company may receive stimulation (shaking, moving or talking) that could stimulate breathing and thus prevent otherwise prolonged post-ictal apnoea.

- **Race.** Afro-American males in the USA carry a higher risk than caucasian males.

- **Medications.** No particular anticonvulsant medication has been associated particularly with SUDEP cases. Drugs such as phenytoin and carbamazepine may affect cardiac conduction, but the practical importance of this is unclear.

- **Alcohol excess.** This appears to be a risk factor for SUDEP.

Mechanisms

SUDEP is a syndrome in which several underlying mechanisms are likely. Studies on a sheep model of induced seizures causing death (Johnston *et al.*, 1997) have helped to clarify the problem.

Central respiratory depression

Apnoea is an almost invariable finding during generalized tonic-clonic seizures (Walker and Fish, 1997); central apnoea occurs in about a third of complex partial seizures. Significant oxygen desaturation may accompany these apnoeas. In the animal model, central apnoea or hypoventilation was the usual cause of death (Johnston *et al.*, 1997).

Pulmonary oedema

A minor degree of pulmonary oedema is common in SUDEP but is not thought to be the actual cause of death. The SUDEP animal model has demonstrated a rise in pulmonary vascular pressure with consequent pulmonary oedema during induced epileptic seizures. The animals that died during an epileptic seizure had much higher pulmonary artery and left atrial pressures than those which survived. The pulmonary oedema was thought to be an effect of both the seizure itself and the seizure-related hypoxaemia rather than being the cause of death.

Cardiac arrhythmia

Cardiac rhythm changes have been well documented in patients with epileptic seizures, both in complex partial and generalized tonic-clonic seizures (Jallon, 1997). The majority of patients develop sinus tachycardia, but occasional patients have bradycardias (Blumhardt *et al.*, 1986).

Supraventricular tachycardia occasionally occurs, but more malignant arrhythmias are unusual. QT interval prolongation may be important in accompanying epileptic activity in susceptible individuals, thus provoking potentially malignant tachyarrhythmias (Tavenor *et al.*, 1996). The influence of anti-epileptic medication on cardiac arrhythmias is unclear. In the animal model, no deaths occurred from malignant tachyarrhythmias. In a case report of a patient who died in a seizure while on video telemetry (Bird, 1997), a pulse artefact is visible on the EEG lead after the cessation of EEG activity, making cardiac arrhythmia unlikely.

QT interval

Prolongation of the QT interval on the ECG is associated with potentially fatal tachyarrhythmias and can occur in a number of situations (*see* Chapter 5). The QT interval is prolonged by intracerebral events including subarachnoid haemorrhage and stroke. Either a shortening or a lengthening of the QT interval may accompany pentylenetetrazol-induced seizures in cats (Lathers and Schraeder, 1982). A relationship between QT prolongation and SUDEP was suggested by Tavenor *et al.* (1996), who found a significant prolongation of the QT interval as assessed on a single ECG channel, accompanying interictal bursts of EEG spike-and-wave 'epileptic' activity. Significant prolongation of the QT interval was seen only in those patients who subsequently succumbed to SUDEP.

Long QT syndromes may cause recurrent blackouts in children, mimicking seizures; should death occur, no post mortem abnormalities are found.

Blood tests for genetic markers of QT interval abnormalities are still possible after death but are currently not routine practice. This may be particularly important because some cases are autosomal dominantly inherited, and other family members, who may also have an erroneous diagnosis of epilepsy, may also be at risk. An ECG is clearly an important investigation in young people with undiagnosed blackouts.

Autonomic variations

Individual normal variations in the autonomic responsiveness of baroreceptors and chemoreceptors (including age-related differences) may determine a difference in susceptibility to apnoea, arrhythmias or blood pressure changes during seizures.

Alcohol

This can influence the anti-epileptic drug level or the seizure threshold and, during a seizure, compromise breathing or enhance the possibility of inhalation.

Genetic factors

Genetic factors may be important, as implied by racial differences in susceptibility.

Differential diagnosis of SUDEP

Patients with SUDEP have, by definition, a normal post mortem examination of the brain and heart, with only minor lung abnormalities. Other conditions causing blackouts diagnosable at autopsy will already have been excluded. Recurrent cardiac arrhythmias, however, such as long QT syndromes, may mimic SUDEP. Arrhythmogenic right ventricular dysplasia and other cardiomyopathies may be missed unless specifically sought.

What to tell patients about SUDEP

Physicians have traditionally rarely raised the subject of sudden unexpected death with patients who have epilepsy. With increasing public and medical awareness of the condition, however, there are grounds to change this practice. Bereaved families of SUDEP victims mostly agree that they would have wished to know about the risk beforehand (Preston, 1997).

Dying during a seizure is an unspoken fear of many people with epilepsy, and a discussion of the facts can at least put this fear into perspective. Discussing SUDEP is difficult for the doctor and patient, and requires a good relationship in order to achieve an open, balanced and trusted discussion tailored to the needs of the individual (Fish, 1997). Written patient information in which the topic of SUDEP is raised is given in an excellent booklet, *Epilepsy in the Young Adult* (Preston, 1998).

When SUDEP is discussed with the patient and carer, emphasis must be placed upon the positive lifestyle measures that may help its prevention:

- Apply **stimulation during witnessed seizures**, for example attending to the patient during seizures in the night and ensuring that he or she is breathing before being left to sleep.
- **Avoid excess alcohol.**
- **Optimize anti-epileptic drug compliance** since minimizing avoidable seizures, particularly generalized tonic-clonic seizures in sleep, seems to be important.

Conclusion

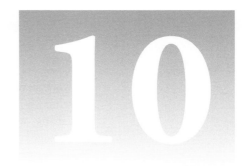

Epilepsy encompasses a broad spectrum of seizure manifestations and severity, its underlying causes being many and varied. The expression of the epilepsies is often age dependent, the problems and approaches to management differing for the neonate, infant, young child, teenager, adult and elderly person. There are also special issues relating to women, especially during their child-bearing years. Many conditions, for example vasovagal syncope and non-epileptic attack disorder, may resemble epilepsy; some conditions, such as panic disorder, frequently co-exist with epilepsy. Correct diagnosis is the basis of epilepsy care, the main route to accurate diagnosis being the clinical history, including a witness account. A syndromic approach to epilepsy diagnosis and an understanding of the differential diagnosis are the keys to its successful management.

The investigation of patients with epilepsy has advanced considerably in recent years. Video EEG now offers physicians the privilege of seeing patients during their attacks. Cerebral imaging provides detailed information on the brain's structure and function, improving our understanding of epilepsy and promoting epilepsy surgery as a potential cure. Genetic studies reveal the rich variety of genetic disorders that may lead to seizures, and several single-gene epilepsy disorders have already been identified. Genetic advances offer considerable promise of a better understanding of epilepsy, as well as real hope for specific and targeted treatments in the future.

The management options for epilepsy continue to develop, particularly with the new range of anti-epileptic medications. Each of the new medications has a broadly similar effectiveness, but they are generally better tolerated than conventional treatments. Epilepsy surgery offers the hope of a cure in selected people. Openness and the provision of information are essential in managing epilepsy. With so much information available to patients, e.g. on the Internet, there is an important need to ensure that the information provided by physicians is accurate, relevant and easily understandable.

Epilepsy commonly involves more than just the neurological disorder. Often prominent are psychiatric associations, social problems relating to stigma, school, work, family interactions, driving privileges and alcohol, learning disabilities, contraception and pregnancy concerns, genetic counselling issues, etc. Because epilepsy crosses specialty boundaries, it is essential that professionals managing epilepsy collaborate and work in teams. Particularly valued is the role of the epilepsy nurse specialist in 'joining up' the service, liaising with primary care and other professionals. Appropriate epilepsy management also frequently involves people other than healthcare professionals, for example social workers and members of voluntary organizations.

Changing people's attitudes towards epilepsy is a major challenge. Doctors should no longer be content with patients having occasional seizures unless several treatment options have first been tried; seizure freedom must be the goal. As we strive to improve the lives of people with epilepsy, we must work towards building more enlightened and tolerant attitudes in society. There is now a real hope of being able to restore and maintain a good quality of life for most patients with epilepsy. The stigma relating to epilepsy, particularly prevalent in underdeveloped countries, will recede as education on the condition broadens. We should increasingly aim towards enabling patients with epilepsy to regain their independence, driving being the only necessarily enforced restriction. We can be hopeful that the progress seen in epilepsy management over the past decade may further allow people with epilepsy increasingly to resume their rightful role in society.

References

Adab, N., Jacoby, A., Smith, D., Chadwick, D.W. 2000 Additional educational needs in children born to mothers with epilepsy. *Journal of Neurology, Neurosurgery and Psychiatry* **68**: 257 (abstract).

Ahmad, D. 2000 WHO to improve epilepsy management in Africa. *Lancet* **355**: 1706.

Aicardi, J. 1996 Myoclonic epilepsies difficult to classify as either Lennox–Gastaut syndrome or myoclonic-astatic epilepsy. In Wallace, S. (ed.) *Epilepsy in children*. London: Chapman & Hall, 271–3.

Alper, K., Devinsky, O., Perrine, K., Vazquez, B., Luciano, D. 1993 Nonepileptic seizures and childhood sexual and physical abuse. *Neurology* **43**: 1950–3.

Aman, M.G., Werry, J.S., Paxton, J.W. *et al*. 1987 Effect of sodium valproate on psychomotor performance in children as a function of dose, fluctuations in concentration, and diagnosis. *Epilepsia* **28**: 115–24.

Annegers, J.F., Hauser, A., Coan, S.P., Rocca, W.A. 1998 A population based study of seizures after traumatic brain injuries. *New England Journal of Medicine* **338**: 20–4.

Appleton, R.E., Chadwick, D., Sweeney, A. 1997 Managing the teenager with epilepsy: paediatric to adult care. *Seizure* **6**: 27–30.

Ballaban-Gil, K., Callahan, C., O'Dell, C., Pappo, M., Moshé, S., Shinnar, S. 1998 Complications of the ketogenic diet. *Epilepsia* **39**: 744–8.

Baraban, S.C., McCarthy, E.B., Schwartzkroin, P.A. 1997 Evidence for increased seizure susceptibility in rats exposed to cocaine in utero. *Brain Research* **102**: 189–96.

Barkovich, A.J., Kuznieeky, R.I., Dobyns, W.B. *et al*. 1996 A classification scheme for malformations of cortical development. *Neuropediatrics* **27**: 59–63.

Ben-David, J., Zipes, D.P. 1993 Torsades de pointes and proarrhythmia. *Lancet* **341**: 1578–82.

Benhorin, J., Medina, A. 1997 Images in medicine. Congenital long-QT syndrome. *New England Journal of Medicine* **336**: 1568.

Berkovic, S.F., Howell, R.A., Hopper, J.L. 1994 Familial temporal lobe epilepsy: a new syndrome with adolescent/adult onset and a benign course. In Wolf P. (ed.) *Epileptic seizures and syndromes*. London: John Libbey, 257–63.

Berkovic, S.F., Scheffer, I.E. 1999 Genetics of the epilepsies. *Current Opinion in Neurology* **12**: 177–82.

Beurs, E de., van Balkom, A.J.L.M., Lange, A., Koele, P., van Dyke, R. 1995 Treatment of panic disorder with agoraphobia: comparison of fluvoxamine, placebo and psychological panic management combined with exposure and of exposure *in vivo* alone. *American Journal of Psychiatry* **152**: 683–91.

Binnie, C.D., MacGillivray, B.B. 1992 Brain mapping – a useful tool or a dangerous toy? *Journal of Neurology, Neurosurgery and Psychiatry* **55**: 527–9.

Bird, J. 1997 Sudden unexplained death in epilepsy: an intracranially monitored case. *Epilepsia* **38**: S52–6.

Blumhardt, L.D., Smith, P.E.M., Owen, L. 1986 Electrocardiographic accompaniments of temporal lobe epileptic seizures. *Lancet* **1**: 1051–6.

Brodie, M.J. 1992 Lamotrigine. *Lancet* **339**: 1397–400.

Brodie, M.J., Biton, V., Montouris, G.D., Shu-Chen 1998 Topiramate therapy in patients with generalized tonic–clonic seizures without focal onset: long-term outcome. *Epilepsia* **39**(suppl. 2): 2 (abstract).

Burn, J., Dennis, M., Bamford, J., Sandercock, P., Wade, D., Warlow, C. 1997 Epileptic seizures after a first stroke: the Oxfordshire community stroke project. *British Medical Journal* **315**: 1582–7.

Camfield, P.R., Camfield, C., Shapiro, S. *et al.* 1980 The first febrile seizure – antipyretic instruction plus either phenobarbital or placebo to prevent a recurrence. *Journal of Pediatrics* **97**: 16–21.

Cavazzutti, G.B. 1980 Epidemiology of different types of epilepsy in school age children of Modena, Italy. *Epilepsia* **21**: 57–62.

Clement, M.J., Wallace, S.J. 1990 Juvenile myoclonic epilepsy. *Archives of Disease in Childhood* **63**: 1049–53.

Cockerell, O.C. 1996 The mortality of epilepsy. *Current Opinion in Neurology* **9**: 93–6.

Cockerell, O.C., Johnson, A.J., Goodridge, D.M.G., Sander, J.W.A.S., Hart, Y.M., Shorvon, S.D. 1994 The mortality of epilepsy: results from the National General Practice Study of Epilepsy. *Lancet* **344**: 918–21.

Cockerell, O.C., Johnson, A.L., Sander, J.W., Hart, Y.M., Shorvon, S.D. 1995 Remission of epilepsy: results from the National General Practice Study of Epilepsy. *Lancet* **346**: 140–4.

Commission on Classification and Terminology of the International League Against Epilepsy 1989 Proposal for revised classification of epilepsies and epileptic syndromes. *Epilepsia* **30**: 389–99.

Consroe, P.F., Wood, G.C., Buchsbaum, H. 1975 Anticonvulsant nature of marihuana smoking. *Journal of the American Medical Association* **234**: 306–7.

Coppola, U., Plouin, P., Chiron, C. *et al.* 1995 Migrating partial seizures in infancy: a malignant disorder with developmental arrest. *Epilepsia* **36**: 1017–24.

Crawford, P.M., Appleton, R., Betts, T., Duncan, J., Guthrie, E., Morrow, J. 1999 Best practice guidelines for the management of women with epilepsy. *Seizure* **8**: 201–17.

Crawford, P.M., West, C.R., Shaw, M.D.M., Chadwick, D.W. 1986 Cerebral arteriovenous malformations and epilepsy: factors in the development of epilepsy. *Epilepsia* **27**: 270–5.

Cummings, L.N., Giudice, L., Morrell, M.J. 1995 Ovulatory function in epilepsy. *Epilepsia* **36**: 355–9.

Dashieff, R.M. 1991 Sudden unexpected death in epilepsy: a series from an epilepsy surgery programme and speculation on the relationship to sudden cardiac death. *Journal of Clinical Neurophysiology* **8**: 216–22.

Davies, J., Smith, P.E.M. 2000 What's in the pipeline for epilepsy patients? *Costs and Options* **20**: 17–19.

Delgado-Escueta, A.V., Greenberg, A.V., Treiman, L. *et al.* 1989 Mapping the gene for juvenile myoclonic epilepsy. *Epilepsia* **30** (suppl. 4), S8–18.

Delgado-Escueta, A.V., Janz, D. 1992 Consensus guidelines: preconception counselling, management and care of the pregnant woman with epilepsy. *Neurology* **42** (suppl. 5): 149–60.

Deshmukh, A., Wittert, W., Schnitzler, E. *et al.* 1986 Lorazepam in the treatment of refractory neonatal seizures. A pilot study. *American Journal of Diseases of Children* **140**: 1042–4.

Dey, A.B., Kenny, R.A. 1997 Drop attacks in the elderly revisited. *Quarterly Journal of Medicine* **90**: 1–3 (editorial).

Dichter, M.A., Brodie, M.J. 1996 New antiepileptic drugs. *New England Journal of Medicine* **334**: 1583–90.

Donaldson, J.O. 1989 Epilepsy. In *Neurology of pregnancy*, 2nd edn. London: W.B. Saunders, 229–67.

Doose, H. 1992 Myoclonic–astatic epilepsy of early childhood. In Roger, J., Dravet, Ch., Bureau, M. *et al.* (eds) *Epileptic syndromes in infancy, childhood and adolescence*, 2nd edn. London: John Libbey, 103–14.

Dravet, Ch., Bureau, M., Roger, J. 1992 Benign myoclonic epilepsy in infants. In Roger, J., Dravet, Ch., Bureau, M. *et al.* (eds) *Epileptic syndromes in infancy, childhood and adolescence*, 2nd edn. London: John Libbey, 67–71.

Dravet, Ch., Genton, P., Bureau, M., Roger, J. 1996 Progressive myoclonus epilepsies. In Wallace, S. (ed.) *Epilepsy in children*. London: Chapman & Hall, 381–93.

DTB 1997 Management of panic disorder. *Drugs and Therapeutics Bulletin* **35**: 58–62.

Duffy, F.H. 1986 Brain electrical activity mapping: ideas and answers. In *Topographic mapping of brain electrical activity*. Boston: Butterworths, 401–98.

Duncan, J. 1997 Positron emission tomography studies of cerebral blood flow and glucose metabolism. *Epilepsia* **38** (suppl. 10): 42–7.

Duncan, J., Panayiotopoulos, C.P. (eds) 1995 *Typical absences and related syndromes*. London: Churchill Livingstone.

Duncan, J., Panayiotopoulos, C.P. (eds) 1996 *Eyelid myoclonia with absences*. London: John Libbey.

Duncan, R. 1997 The clinical use of SPECT in focal epilepsy. *Epilepsia* **38** (suppl. 10): 39–41.

Duncan, S., Read, C.L., Brodie, M.J. 1993 How common is catamenial epilepsy? *Epilepsia* **34**: 827–31.

Edeh, J., Toone, B. 1987 Relationship between interictal psychopathology and the type of epilepsy. Results of a survey in general practice. *British Journal of Psychiatry* **151**: 95–101.

Eke, T., Talbot, J.F., Lawden, M.C. 1997 Severe persistent visual field constriction associated with vigabatrin. *British Medical Journal* **314**: 180–1.

Elia, M., Guerrini, R., Musumeci, S.A. *et al.* 1998 Myoclonic absence-like seizures and chromosome abnormality syndromes. *Epilepsia* **39**: 660–3.

Elmazar, M.M.A., Thiel, R., Nau, H. 1992 Effect of supplementation with folinic acid, vitamin B_6 and vitamin B_{12} on valproic acid induced teratogenesis in mice. *Fundamental and Applied Toxicology* **18**: 389–94.

Elmslie, F., Gardiner, M. 1995 Genetics of the epilepsies. *Current Opinion in Neurology* **8**: 126–9.

Feely, M., Calvert, R., Gibson, J. 1982. Clobazam in catamenial epilepsy: a model for evaluating anticonvulsants. *Lancet* **2**: 71–3.

Fish, D.R. 1995 The role of encephalography. In Hopkins, A., Shorvon, S., Cascino, G. (eds) *Epilepsy*, 2nd edn. London: Chapman & Hall, 123–42.

Fish, D.R. 1997 Sudden unexpected death in epilepsy: impact on clinical practice. *Epilepsia* **38** (suppl.11): S60–2.

Fish, D.R., Quirk, J.A., Smith, S.J.M. *et al.* 1994 *National survey of photosensitivity and seizures induced by electronic screen games*. London: Department of Trade and Industry.

Gaily, E., Granstrom, M.-L. 1992 Minor abnormalities in children of mothers with epilepsy. *Neurology* **42**: 128–31.

Garcia, H.H., Gilman, R., Martinez, M. *et al.* 1993 Cysticercosis as a major cause of epilepsy in Peru. The Cysticercosis Working Group in Peru (CWG). *Lancet* **341**: 197–200.

Gates, J.R., Luciano, D., Devinsky, O. 1991. The classification and treatment of nonepileptic events. In Devinsky, O., Theodore, W.H. (eds) *Epilepsy and behavior*. New York: Wiley-Liss, 251–63.

Gilham, R.A., Blacklaw, J., McKee, P.J. *et al.* 1993 Effect of vigabatrin on sedation and cognitive function in patients with refractory epilepsy. *Journal of Neurology, Neurosurgery and Psychiatry* **56**: 1271–5.

Handforth, A., DeGiorgio, C.M., Schachter, S.C. *et al.* 1998 Vagus nerve stimulation therapy for partial-onset seizures: a randomized active-control trial. *Neurology* **51**: 48–55.

Harding, G.F.A., Jeavons, P.M. 1994 *Photosensitive epilepsy*, London: MacKeith Press.

Hart, Y.M., Sander, J.W.A.S., Johnson, A.L., Shorvon, S.D. 1990 National General Practice Study of Epilepsy: recurrence after a first seizure. *Lancet* **336**: 1271–4.

Hashimoto, K., Fujita, T., Furuja, M. *et al.* 1989 Absence seizures following febrile seizures. *Brain & Development* **11**: 268.

Hauser, W.A., Annegers, J.F. 1993 Epidemiology of epilepsy. In Laidlaw, J., Richens, A., Chadwick, D.W. (eds) *A textbook of epilepsy*. Edinburgh: Churchill Livingstone, 23–45.

Hauser, W.A., Annegers, J.F., Rocca, W.A. 1996 Descriptive epidemiology of epilepsy: contributions of population-based studies from Rochester, Minnesota. *Mayo Clinic Proceedings* **71**: 576–86.

Hellström-Westas, L., Westgren, U., Rosn, I. *et al.* 1988 Lidocaine for treatment of severe seizures in newborn infants. I Clinical effects and cerebral electrical activity monitoring during intravenous infusion. *Acta Paediatrica Scandinavica* **77**: 79–84.

Herzog, A.G. 1995 Progesterone therapy in women with complex partial and secondary generalized seizures. *Neurology* **45**: 1660–2.

Howe, A.M., Lipson, A.H., Sheffield, L.J. *et al.* 1995 Prenatal exposure to phenytoin, facial development, and a possible role for vitamin K. *American Journal of Medical Genetics* **58**: 238–44.

Howell, S.J.L., Owen, L., Chadwick, D.W. 1989 Pseudostatus epilepticus. *Quarterly Journal of Medicine* **266**: 507–19.

Hummel, C., Stefan, H. 1997 Magnetoencephalography. *Epilepsia* **38** (suppl. 10): 52–7.

ILAE Neuroimaging Commission 1997 ILAE Neuroimaging Commission recommendations for neuroimaging of patients with epilepsy. *Epilepsia* **38** (suppl. 10): 1–2.

Isojarvi, J.I.T., Laatikainen, T.J., Pakarinen, A.J., Juntunen, K.T.S., Myllyla, V.V. 1993 Polycystic ovaries and hyperandrogenism in women taking valproate for epilepsy. *New England Journal of Medicine* **329**: 1383–8.

Jallon, P. 1997 Arrhythmogenic seizures. *Epilepsia* **38** (suppl.11): S43–7.

Johnston, S.C., Siedenberg, R., Min, J.K., Jerome, E.H., Laxer, K.D. 1997 Central apnea and acute cardiac ischemia in a sheep model of epileptic sudden death. *Annals of Neurology* **42**: 588–94.

Kale, R. 1998 The treatment gap in epilepsy. *World Neurology* **12**: 11.

Kalviainen, R., Aikia, M., Partanen, J. *et al.* 1991 Randomized controlled study of vigabatrin versus carbamazepine monotherapy in newly diagnosed patients with epilepsy: an interim report. *Journal of Child Neurology* **6**: 560–9.

Kilpatrick, C.J., Davis, S.M., Tress, B.M. *et al.* 1990 Epileptic seizures in acute stroke. *Archives of Neurology* **47**: 157–60.

Koch, S., Loesche, G., Jager-Roman, E. *et al.* 1992 Major birth malformations and antiepileptic drugs. *Neurology* **42** (S5): 83–8.

Lamoureux, D., Spencer, S.S. 1995 Epilepsy surgery in adults. *Current Opinion in Neurology* **8**: 107–11.

Lancet 1991 Teratogenesis with carbamazepine. *Lancet* **337**: 1316–17 (editorial).

Lathers, C.M., Schraeder, P.L. 1982 Autonomic dysfunction in epilepsy: characterization of autonomic cardiac neural discharge associated with pentylenetetrazol-induced epileptogenic activity. *Epilepsia* **23**: 633–47.

Leach, J.P., Brodie, M.J. 1998 Tiagabine. *Lancet* **351**: 203–7.

Leach, J.P., Marson, A., Hutton, J., Chadwick, D.W. 1999 A meta-analysis of the efficacy and tolerability of remacemide in clinical studies. *Epilepsia* **40**: 145 (abstract).

Lempert, T., Bauer, M., Schmidt, D. 1994 Syncope: a videometric analysis of 56 episodes of transient cerebral hypoxia. *Annals of Neurology* **36**: 233–7.

Li, L.M., Fish, D.R., Sisodiya, S.M., Shorvon, S.D., Alsanjhari, N., Stevens, J.M. 1995 High resolution magnetic resonance imaging in adults with partial or secondary generalized epilepsy attending a tertiary referral unit. *Journal of Neurology, Neurosurgery and Psychiatry* **59**: 384–7.

Loiseau, P. 1992 Childhood absence epilepsy. In Bureau, M., Roger, J., Dravet, Ch. *et al.* (eds) *Epileptic syndromes in infancy, childhood and adolescence*, 2nd edn. London: John Libbey, 135–50.

Lundorf, K., Jensen, L.D., Plesner, A.M. 1986 Etiology of seizures in the elderly. *Epilepsia* **27**: 458–64.

McAreavey, M.J., Ballinger, B.R., Fenton, G.W. 1992 Epileptic seizures in elderly patients with dementia. *Epilepsia* **33**: 647–60.

McCrory, P.R., Bladin, P.F., Berkovic, S.F. 1997 Retrospective study of concussive convulsions in elite Australian rules and rugby league footballers: phenomenology, aetiology and outcome. *British Medical Journal* **314**: 171–4.

Manford, M., Hart, Y.M., Sander, J.W., Shorvon, S.D. 1992 The National General Practice Study of Epilepsy: the syndromic classification of the International League Against Epilepsy applied to epilepsy in a general population. *Archives of Neurology* **49**: 801–9.

Manonmani, V., Wallace, S.J. 1994 Epilepsy with myoclonic absences. *Archives of Disease in Childhood* **70**: 288–90.

Manuchehri, K., Goodman, S., Siviter, L., Nightingale, S. 2000 A controlled study of vigabatrin and visual abnormalities. *British Journal of Ophthalmology* **84**: 499–505.

Marks, W.J., Laxer, K.D. 1998 Semiology of temporal lobe seizures: value in lateralizing the seizure focus. *Epilepsia* **39**: 721–6.

Marson, A.G., Kadir, Z.A., Chadwick, D.W. 1996 New antiepileptic drugs: a systematic review of their efficacy and tolerability. *British Medical Journal* **313**: 1169–74.

Mathews, B. 1975 Epilepsy. In *Practical neurology.* London: Blackwell Scientific Publications, 48–75.

Mattson, R.H., Cramer, J.A., Darney, P.D., Naftolin, F. 1986 Use of oral contraceptives by women with epilepsy. *Journal of the American Medical Association* **256**: 238–40.

Meencke, H.J., Janz, D. 1984 Neuropathological findings in primary generalized epilepsy: a study of eight cases. *Epilepsia* **25**: 8–21.

MRC (Medical Research Council Antiepileptic Drug Withdrawal Study Group) 1991a Randomised study of antiepileptic drug withdrawal in patients in remission. *Lancet* **337**: 1175–80.

MRC (Medical Research Council Vitamin Study Research Group) 1991b Prevention of neural-tube defects: results of the Medical Research Council Vitamin Study. *Lancet* **338**: 131–7.

Nagao, H., Morimoto, T., Takahashi, M. *et al.* 1990 The circadian rhythm of typical absence seizures – the frequency and duration of paroxysmal discharges. *Neuropediatrics* **21**: 79–82.

Naidu, S., Niedermeyer, E. 1993 Degenerative disorders of the central nervous system In Niedermeyer, E., Lopes da Silva, F. (eds) *Electroencephalography: basic principles, clinical applications and related fields,* 3rd edn. Baltimore: Williams & Wilkins, 351–71.

Nashef, L. 1997 Sudden unexpected death in epilepsy: terminology and definitions. *Epilepsia* **38** (suppl.11): S6–8.

Nashef, L., Fish, D.R., Sander, J.W.A.S., Shorvon, S.D. 1995 Incidence of sudden unexpected death in an adult outpatient cohort at a tertiary referral centre. *Journal of Neurology, Neurosurgery and Psychiatry* **58**: 462–4.

Nashef, L., Walker, F., Allen, P., Sander, J.W., Shorvon, S.D., Fish, D.R. 1996 Apnoea and bradycardia during epileptic seizures: relation to sudden unexpected death in epilepsy. *Journal of Neurology, Neurosurgery and Psychiatry* **60**: 297–300.

Neubauer, B.S., Fiedler, B., Himmelein, B. *et al.* 1998 Centrotemporal spikes in families with benign rolandic epilepsy: linkage to chromosome 15q 14. *Neurology* **51**: 1608–12.

Nielsen, J.P. 1995 Magnesium sulphate: the drug of choice in eclampsia. *British Medical Journal* **311**: 702–3.

Ohtahara, S., Ohtsuka, Y., Yamatogi, Y. *et al.* 1987 The early infantile epileptic encephalopathy with suppression-burst: developmental aspects. *Brain & Development* **9**: 371–6.

Okumura, A., Hayakawa, F., Kuno, K. *et al.* 1996 Benign partial epilepsy in infancy. *Archives of Disease in Childhood* **74**: 19–21.

Oldani, A., Zucconi, M., Asselta, R. *et al.* 1998 Autosomal dominant nocturnal frontal lobe epilepsy. *Brain* **121**: 205–23.

Omtzigt, J.G.C., Los, F.J., Grobee, D.E. *et al.* 1992 The risk of spina bifida aperta after first-trimester exposure to valproate in a prenatal cohort. *Neurology* **42**(S5): 119–25.

Opeskin, K., Burke, M.P., Cordner, S.M., Berkovic, S.F. 1999 Comparison of antiepileptic drug levels in sudden unexpected deaths in epilepsy with deaths from other causes. *Epilepsia* **40**: 1795–8.

Panayiotopoulos, C.P. 1994 Elementary visual hallucinations in migraine and epilepsy. *Journal of Neurology, Neurosurgery and Psychiatry*, **57**: 1371–4.

Panayiotopoulos, C.P. 1996 Juvenile myoclonic epilepsy. In Wallace, S. (ed.) *Epilepsy in children.* London: Chapman & Hall, 333–47.

Panayiotopoulos, C.P. 1999 *Benign childhood partial seizures and related epileptic syndromes.* London: John Libbey.

Panayiotopoulos, C.P., Ferrie, C.D., Giannakodimos, S.E. *et al.* 1994 Perioral myoclonia with absences: a new syndrome. In Wolf, P. (ed.) *Epileptic seizures and syndromes.* London: John Libbey, 143–53.

Penry, J.K., Porter, R.J., Dreifuss, F.E. 1975 Simultaneous recording of absence seizures with video tape and electroencephalography. A study of 374 seizures in 48 patients. *Brain* **98**: 427–40.

Plouin, P., Dulac, O. 1994 Other types of seizures. In Dulac, O., Chugani, H.T., Dalla Bernardino, B. (eds) *Infantile spasms and West syndrome.* London: W.B. Saunders, 52–62.

Preston, J. 1997 Information on sudden deaths from epilepsy. *Epilepsia* **38** (suppl.11): S72–4.

Preston, J. 1998 *Epilepsy and the young adult.* London: EYA.

Robinson, J.R., Awad, I.A., Little, J.R. 1991 Natural history of the cavernous angioma. *Journal of Neurosurgery* **75**: 709–14.

Rocca, W.A., Sharbrough, T.W., Hauser, W.A. *et al.* 1987 Risk factors for absence seizures: a population-based case-control study in Rochester, Minnesota. *Neurology* **37**: 1309–14.

Ronen, G.M., Rosales, T.D., Connolly, M. *et al.* 1993 Seizure characteristics in chromosome 20 benign familial neonatal convulsions. *Neurology* **43**: 1355–60.

Rosa, F.L.O. 1991 Spina bifida in infants of women treated with carbamazepine during pregnancy. *New England Journal of Medicine* **324**: 674–7.

Sander, J.W., Hart, Y.M., Johnson, A.L., Shorvon, S.D. 1990 National General Practice Study of Epilepsy: newly diagnosed epileptic seizures in a general population. *Lancet* **338**: 1267–71.

Sander, J.W.A.S., Shorvon, S.D. 1996 Epidemiology of the epilepsies. *Journal of Neurology, Neurosurgery and Psychiatry* **61**: 433–43.

Scambler, G. 1998 Stigma and disease: changing paradigms. *Lancet* **352**: 1054–5.

Schachter, S.C., Saper, C.B. 1998 Vagus nerve stimulation. *Epilepsia* **39**: 677–86.

Scheffer, I.E., Berkovic, S.F. 1997 Generalized epilepsy with febrile seizures plus. A genetic disorder with heterogeneous clinical phenotypes. *Brain* **120**: 479–90.

Scheffer, I.E., Bhatia, K.P., Lopes-Cendes, I. *et al.* 1995 Autosomal dominant nocturnal frontal lobe epilepsy. A distinctive clinical disorder. *Brain* **118**: 61–73.

Scher, M.S., Aso, K., Beggarly, M.E. *et al.* 1993 Electrographic seizures in pre-term and full-term neonates: clinical correlates, associated brain lesions, and risks for neurologic sequelae. *Pediatrics* **91**: 128–34.

Scheure, M.L. 1995 Seizures and epilepsy in the elderly. In Pedley, T.A., Meldrum, B.S. (eds) *Recent advances in epilepsy.* Edinburgh: Churchill Livingstone, 247–70.

Schierhout, G., Roberts, I. 1998 Prophylactic antiepileptic agents after head injury: a systematic review. *Journal of Neurology, Neurosurgery and Psychiatry* **64**: 108–12.

Schupf, N., Ottoman, R. 1994 Likelihood of pregnancy in individuals with idiopathic/cryptogenic epilepsy: social and biologic influence. *Epilepsia* **35**: 750–6.

Scott, R.C., Besag, F.M., Neville, B.G. 1999 Buccal midazolam and rectal diazepam for treatment of prolonged seizures in childhood and adolescence: a randomised trial. *Lancet* **353**: 1371–4.

Sheth, R., Wesolowski, C., Jacob, J., Penney, S., Hobbs, G., Riggs, J., Bodensteiner, J. 1995 Effect of carbamazepine and valproate on bone mineral density. *Journal of Pediatrics* **127**: 256–62.

Shorvon, S. 1994 *Status epilepticus: its clinical features and treatment in children and adults.* Cambridge: Cambridge University Press.

Shorvon, S.D. 1995 The classic genetics of the epilepsies. In Hopkins, A., Shorvon, S., Cascino, G. (eds) *Epilepsy*, 2nd edn. London: Chapman & Hall Medical, 87–92.

Shorvon, S. 2000 Levetiracetam. In *Handbook of epilepsy treatment.* Oxford: Blackwell Science, 113–16.

Singh, B., Al Shahwan, S.A., Habbab, M.A., Al Deeb, S.M., Biary, N. 1993 Idiopathic long QT syndrome: asking the right question. *Lancet* **341**: 741–2.

Sisodiya, S.M. 2000 Surgery for malformations of cortical development causing epilepsy. *Brain* **123**: 1075–91.

Smith, D.W., Jones, K.L. 1996 *Recognizable patterns of human malformation: genetics, embryologic and clinical aspects.* Philadelphia: W.B. Saunders.

Smith, P.E.M. 1998 The teenager with epilepsy. *British Medical Journal* **317**: 960–1.

Smith, P.E.M., McBride, A. 1999 Illicit drugs and seizures. *Seizure* **8**: 441–3 (editorial).

Smith, P.E.M., Saunders, J., Dawson, A., Kerr, M.P. 1999 Intractable seizures in pregnancy. *Lancet* **354**: 1522.

Spitz, M.C., Towbin, J.A., Shantz, D., Adler, L.E. 1995 Risk factors for burns as a consequence of seizures in persons with epilepsy. *Epilepsia* **35**: 764–7.

Stroink, H., Brouwer, O.F., Arts, W.F. *et al.* 1998 The first unprovoked, untreated seizure in childhood: a hospital based study of the accuracy of the diagnosis, rate of recurrence, and long term outcome after recurrence. Dutch study of epilepsy in childhood. *Journal of Neurology, Neurosurgery and Psychiatry* **64**: 595–600.

Sveinbjornsdottir, S., Duncan, J. 1993 Parietal and occipital lobe epilepsy: a review. *Epilepsia* **34**: 493–521.

Tallis, R. 1995 *Epilepsy in elderly people.* London: Martin Dunitz.

Tassinari, C.A., Bureau, M., Thomas, P. 1992 Epilepsy with myoclonic absences. In Roger, J., Bureau, M., Dravet, Ch., Dreifuss, F.E., Perrett, A., Wolf, P. (eds) *Epileptic syndromes in infancy, childhood and adolescence.* London: John Libbey, 151–60.

Tavenor, S.J., Brown, S.W., Tavenor, R.M.E., Gifford, C. 1996 Electrocardiograph QT lengthening associated with epileptiform electro-encephalographic discharges – a role in sudden unexpected death in epilepsy? *Seizure* **5**: 79–83

Taylor, D.C. 1996 Psychiatric aspects. In Wallace, S.J. (ed.) *Epilepsy in children.* London: Chapman & Hall, 601–16.

Taylor, J., Chadwick, D.W., Johnson, T. 1995 Accident experience and notification rates in people with recent seizures, epilepsy or undiagnosed episodes of loss of consciousness. *Quarterly Journal of Medicine* **88**: 733–40.

Tennis, P., Cole, T.B., Annegers, J.F., Leestma, J.E., McNutt, M., Rajput, A. 1995 Cohort study of incidence of sudden unexplained death in persons with seizure disorder treated with antiepileptic drugs in Saskatchewan, Canada. *Epilepsia* **36**: 29–36.

Trimble, M.R. 1991 *The psychoses of epilepsy.* New York: Raven Press.

Viskin, S. 1999 Long QT syndromes and torsade de pointes. *Lancet* **354**: 1625–33.

Volpe, J.J. 1995 Neonatal seizures. In *Neurology of the newborn*, 3rd edn. Philadelphia: W. B. Saunders, 172–207.

Walker, F., Fish, D.R. 1997 Recording respiratory parameters in patients with epilepsy. *Epilepsia* **38** (suppl.11): S41–2.

Wallace, S.J. 1996 Electroencephalography. In Wallace, S.J. (ed.) *Epilepsy in children.* London: Chapman & Hall, 451–70.

Wallace, S.J. 2000 Which anticonvulsant? *Current Paediatrics* **10**: 28–32.

Walsh, C.A. 1999 Genetic malformations of the human cerebral cortex. *Neuron* **23**: 19–29.

Wilkins, A., Lindsay, J. 1985 Common forms of reflex epilepsy: physiological mechanisms and techniques for treatment. In Pedley, T.A., Meldrum,

B.S. (eds) *Recent advances in epilepsy*, vol. 2. Edinburgh: Churchill Livingstone, 239–71.

Wills, A.J., Stevens, D.L. 1994 Epilepsy in the accident and emergency department. *British Journal of Hospital Medicine* **52**: 42–5.

Woermann, F.G., Free, S.L., Koepp, M.J., Sisodiya, S.M., Duncan, J.S. 1999 Abnormal cerebral structure in juvenile myoclonic epilepsy demonstrated with voxel-based analysis of MRI. *Brain* **122**: 2101–8.

Wolf, P. 1992 Juvenile myoclonic epilepsy. In Roger, J., Bureau, M., Dravet, Ch. *et al.* (eds) *Epileptic syndromes in infancy, childhood and adolescence.* London: John Libbey, 313–28.

Wolf, P., Gooses, R. 1986 Relation of photosensitivity to epileptic syndromes. *Journal of Neurology, Neurosurgery and Psychiatry,* **49**: 1386–91.

Yerby, M.S., Friel, P.N., McCormick, K.B. *et al.* 1990 Pharmacokinetics of anticonvulsants in pregnancy: alterations in plasma protein binding. *Epilepsy Research* **5**: 223–8.

Further reading

Aicardi, J. 1988 *Diseases of the nervous system in childhood*, 2nd edn. Cambridge: MacKeith Press.

Engel, J., Pedley, T.A. (eds) 1997 *Epilepsy. A comprehensive textbook*. Philadelphia: Lippincott-Raven.

Hopkins, A., Shorvon, S., Cascino, G. (eds) 1995 *Epilepsy*, 2nd edn. London: Chapman & Hall Medical.

Kotagal, P., Lüders, H. 1999 *The epilepsies. Etiologies and prevention*. San Diego: Academic Press.

Shorvon, S. 1994 *Status epilepticus: its clinical features and treatment in children and adults*. Cambridge: Cambridge University Press.

Shorvon, S. 2000 *Handbook of epilepsy treatment*. Oxford: Blackwell Science.

Wallace, S.J. 1996 *Epilepsy in children*. London: Chapman & Hall.

Useful addresses

National Society for Epilepsy
Chalfont St Peter
Gerrards Cross
Buckinghamshire
SL9 0RJ
UK
Tel: 01494 601300
Helpline: 01494 601400

British Epilepsy Association
New Anstey House
Gate Way Drive
Yeadon
Leeds
LS19 7XY
UK
Tel: 0113 2108800
Helpline: 0808 8005050
E-mail: epilepsy@bea.org.uk
Website: www.epilepsy.org.uk
(Useful patient information about
epilepsy is available on the BEA
website.)

Epilepsy Association of Scotland
48 Govan Road
Glasgow
G51 1JL
Tel: 0141 419 1701
Helpline: 0141 427 5225
Website:
www.epilepsyscotland.org.uk

Epilepsy Wales/Epilepsi Cymru
15 Chester Street
St Asaph
Denbighshire
LL17 0RE
Helpline: 0345 413774

Index